The Prostate Cancer Protection Plan

Also by Robert Arnot, M.D.

The Best Medicine

Dr. Bob Arnot's Guide to Turning Back the Clock

Dr. Bob Arnot's Revolutionary Weight Control Program

The Breast Cancer Prevention Diet

The Biology of Success

with Charles Gaines

Sportselection

Sportstalent

The Prostate Cancer Protection Plan

The Powerful Foods, Supplements, and Drugs That Could Save Your Life

Robert Arnot, M.D.

LITTLE, BROWN AND COMPANY

Boston New York London

This book is not intended as a substitute for medical advice of physicians. The reader should regularly consult a physician in all matters relating to his or her health, and particularly in respect of any symptoms that may require diagnosis or medical attention.

First Edition

Library of Congress Cataloging-in-Publication Data
Arnot, Robert Burns.
    The prostate cancer protection plan: the powerful foods, supplements, and drugs that could save your life / Robert Arnot.
        p.   cm.
    Includes bibliographical references and index.
    ISBN 0-316-05153-5
    1. Prostate — Cancer — Diet therapy. I. Title.
RC280.P7 A764 2000
616.99'463 — dc21   00-025751

10   9   8   7   6   5   4   3   2   1

Q-FG

Designed by Joyce Weston
Printed in the United States of America

To my dear grandfather,
Patrick "P. J." Burns, who was
beloved by all who knew him

Contents

Acknowledgments

A book of this scope and magnitude rides on the shoulders of hundreds of determined researchers, doctors, and patients who have made enormous contributions toward the day when prostate cancer will be conquered. In particular, I offer my profound thanks and gratitude to the following people for their dedication and for the countless hours they were willing to give to make this a better book.

Peter Albertsen, M.D., at the University of Connecticut Health Center.

Atif Awad, Ph.D., R.D., Associate Professor and Director of Nutrition at the State University of New York at Buffalo.

Stephen Barnes, Ph.D., Professor of Pharmacology, Toxicology, Biochemistry, and Molecular Genetics at the University of Alabama at Birmingham School of Medicine.

Otis Brawley, M.D., at the National Cancer Institute.

James Brooks, M.D., Associate Chief of Urologic Oncology at Stanford University.

Ralph Buttyan, Ph.D., Professor and Director of Urology Research at Columbia University.

William Catalona, M.D., Professor of Urology at Washington University School of Medicine in St. Louis.

June Chan, Sc.D., Postdoctoral Research Fellow at the Harvard School of Public Health.

Sophie Chen, Ph.D., Director of NovaSpes Research Laboratory and Research Associate Professor of Medicine at New York Medical College.

Steven K. Clinton, M.D., Ph.D., Professor at the Ohio State University Health Sciences Center.

John Codington, Ph.D., at the Boston Biomedical Research Institute.

Donald Coffey, Ph.D., Professor of Oncology, Urology, Pharmacology and Molecular Sciences, and Pathology at Johns Hopkins University.

George Comstock, M.D., at Johns Hopkins University.

E. David Crawford, M.D., Professor of Surgery (Urology) and Radiation Oncology at the University of Colorado Health Sciences Center.

Bill Donnelly, prostate cancer survivor.

Bob Each, prostate cancer survivor.

Ronald Evans, Ph.D., at the Salk Institute in San Diego.

David Feldman, M.D., Professor of Medicine at Stanford University.

Neil Fleshner, M.D., Urologic Oncologist at the University of Toronto.

Ivan Flowers, prostate cancer survivor.

Jeffrey Forman, M.D., Professor of Radiation Oncology at Wayne State University in Detroit.

Richard Gallager, Ph.D., Epidemiologist at the University of Vancouver.

K. Dun Gifford, President and Founder of Oldways Preservation Trust.

John Gohagain, Ph.D., at the National Cancer Institute.

Erik Goluboff, M.D., Assistant Professor of Urology at Columbia University and Director of Urology at the Allen Pavilion of Columbia-Presbyterian Medical Center.

David Grignon, M.D., at Wayne State University in Detroit.

Richard Hayes, Ph.D., of the National Cancer Institute.

David Heber, M.D., at the Center for Human Nutrition at the University of California in Los Angeles.

Warren Heston, M.D., at Sloan-Kettering Hospital.

Kenneth V. Honn, Ph.D., Professor of Radiation Oncology and Pathology at Wayne State University in Detroit, and Director of the Prostate Cancer Program at the Karmanos Cancer Institute.

Anne Hsing, Ph.D., Epidemiologist at the National Cancer Institute.

Steven Hursting, Ph.D., M.P.H., at the University of Texas M. D. Anderson Cancer Center.

William Isaacs, Ph.D., Professor of Urology at Johns Hopkins University.

Philip Kantoff, M.D., at the Dana-Farber Cancer Institute in Boston.

Frank W. Kerry, Ph.D., toxicologist at the National Institute of Environemental Health Sciences (NIEHS).

Laurence Kolonel, M.D., Ph.D., Professor at the University of Hawaii.

Barnett Kramer, M.D., M.P.H., at the National Cancer Institute.

Robert Krane, M.D., Director of Neurology at Massachusetts General Hospital.

Alan Kristal, Ph.D., Epidemiologist at the Fred Hutchinson Cancer Center in Seattle.

Fred Lee, M.D., at the Crittenton Hospital in Rochester, Michigan.

Nancy Lightfoot, Ph.D., Director of Epidemiology at the Northeastern Ontario Regional Cancer Center.

Christopher Logothetis, M.D., at the University of Texas M. D. Anderson Cancer Center.

John McDougal, M.D., at St. Helena Hospital in Napa Valley, California.

Bruce McEwen, Ph.D., Professor of Neuroendocrinology at Rockefeller University.

Gail McKeown-Eyssen, Ph.D., Professor of Epidemiology at the University of Toronto.

Curtis Mettlin, Ph.D., Epidemiologist at the Roswell Park Cancer Institute in Buffalo, New York.

François Meyer, M.D., Ph.D., Professor at Laval University.

Michael Milken, Founder and Chairman of the Association for the Cure of Cancer of the Prostate (CaP CURE).

Charles Myers, M.D., Director of the Cancer Center at the University of Virginia.

Linda Nebeling, Ph.D., M.P.H., R.D., Nutritionist at the National Cancer Institute.

William Nelson, M.D., Ph.D., Medical Oncologist at Johns Hopkins University.

Abraham Nomura, Ph.D, Professor at the University of Hawaii.

Carl A. Olsson, M.D., Professor and Chairman of Urology at Columbia University.

Dean Ornish, M.D., preventive medicine pioneer.

Rifat Pamukcu, Ph.D., of Cell Pathways Inc.

Gary Pasternak, M.D., Ph.D., Molecular Pathologist at Johns Hopkins University.

Daniel Petrylak, M.D., at Columbia University.

Kenneth J. Pienta, M.D., Professor of Internal Medicine at the University of Michigan.

Harry Pinchot, prostate cancer survivor.

Ronald K. Ross, M.D., Chairman of the Department of Preventive Medicine at the University of Southern California.

Enrike Saez, Ph.D., at the Salk Institute in San Diego.

Wael Sakr, M.D., Associate Professor of Pathology at Wayne State University in Detroit.

George Salazar, prostate cancer survivor.

Joseph Schmidt, M.D., Professor of Urology at the University of California in San Diego.

Jonathan Simons, M.D., Associate Professor of Oncology and Urology at Johns Hopkins University.

Eric Small, M.D., Professor of Medicine and Urology at the University of California in San Francisco.

Janet Stanford, Ph.D., at the Fred Hutchinson Cancer Center.

Sarah Strom, Ph.D., of the University of Texas M. D. Anderson Cancer Center.

Paul Talalay, M.D., Professor of Pharmacology and Molecular Sciences at Johns Hopkins University.

Donald L. Trump, M.D., Chief of Hematology/Oncology and Professor of Medicine and Surgery at the University of Pittsburgh School of Medicine.

Milan Uskokovic, Ph.D., world's leading expert on 1,25 analogs, and consultant to Hoffmann La Roche.

Howard Waage, prostate cancer survivor.

Patrick Walsh, M.D., Professor and Director of Urology at Johns

Hopkins University and Director of the James Buchanan Brady Urological Institute at the Johns Hopkins Hospital.

Alice Whittemore, Ph.D., Health Research and Policies Professor at Stanford University.

Walter Willett, M.D., Professor at the Harvard School of Public Health.

David Wood, M.D, Professor of Urology at Wayne State University in Detroit.

Robert Yannone, prostate cancer survivor.

I'd like to thank the following members of the team who made this book possible:

Rima Canaan, my research and editorial colleague, who doggedly pursued thousands of leads and interviewed hundreds of doctors and patients in pursuit of the truth. I'd like to thank her for her determined effort to make this a far better book through her unflagging quest for excellence.

Bill Phillips, my editor, who devoted hundreds of hours to help sharpen and crystallize the central themes of this book. He's one of a rare surviving breed of phenomenal editors whose sharp eye and creative vision take the ordinary and transform it into the extraordinary.

Betty Power, my copyeditor, who worked heroically and exhaustively to make this book come together. Her effort, zeal, and enthusiasm are to be highly commended.

Sarah Crichton, my publisher, who had the vision to foresee the tremendous importance of cancer prevention. Her enthusiastic backing, charm, and leadership are largely responsible for the success of this book.

Larry Kirshbaum, the president of Time Warner Trade Publishing, who instinctively knew the importance of protecting men against prostate cancer and backed this book from the beginning. His charismatic leadership has been an inspiration and a joy to all of us who've had the honor of working with him.

Simon and Dan Green, my agents, who for over a decade have helped to shape and transform my career as a writer.

The Prostate Cancer Protection Plan

Introduction

There's nothing I look forward to more than starting a fresh new day. That wasn't always the case. I used to drag myself out of bed and limp through the first part of the morning wondering why I had ever gotten up. (I hope the people I worked for weren't thinking the same thing!) But now, when I go to sleep, I can barely contain my enthusiasm for what the morning will bring. What's made the difference? A remarkable new diet. One that makes me lean and energetic, gives me great stamina and a tremendously positive mental attitude. It's literally changed my life. I start each morning with a special soy protein shake. Minutes after downing my drink, the last shadows of sleepiness have vanished because of a special ingredient called tyrosine. I become alive again, brimming with mental energy and physical vigor. That powers me through an hour on the stair machine and 30 minutes of yoga. I follow that with whole-grain, high-fiber cereal, berries, and half a cantaloupe, all of which give me sustained energy through the morning without the crash and burn you may find with coffee and bagels. I've given up the soporific pasta lunch for a black bean burrito with vegetables. They're among the dozens of wonderful new foods and meals I've learned to love.

What brought about the change? I can only credit my wife. It all goes back to a simple question she asked me. You see, her mother developed breast cancer at a strikingly young age. My wife, naturally concerned about her risk of cancer, asked me what she might do to prevent getting breast cancer herself. Like most physicians, I answered by reflex: "There's nothing you can do." But my wife then threw down the gauntlet. She said: "You're a doctor, you're a journalist, you figure it out."

I took her challenge, traveling far and wide to see what might influence her chances of breast cancer. I was fascinated to find time and again that the clues led to nutrition as the fuel that causes many breast cancers to grow. As my wife and I looked for the powerful foods and supplements that might actually prevent breast cancer, the idea of writing a book for my wife, Courtney, and her friends was born. It was published in 1998 under the title *The Breast Cancer Prevention Diet*. It clearly struck a nerve. It became number one on the Amazon.com, *New York Times,* and *Wall Street Journal* bestseller lists. Women still stop me on the street and thank me for writing it. I am grateful to all of these women for their kindness and brave spirit, but their gratitude is better placed at the feet of those courageous women who volunteered to participate in many of the research studies that tested nutrition as a way to prevent cancer. Sure, there are other ways of lowering the risk of breast cancer. There are powerful new drugs already proven to be effective in rigorous clinical trials. Oncologists believe that as many as 28 million women should consider them. However, whenever I lecture on breast cancer, I poll the audience. I ask them, "How many of you would take a drug to prevent breast cancer?" At best four or five women raise their hands in an audience of nearly three hundred women. When I ask how many would cast their lot with a change in diet, a sea of hands is raised. I still urge women to carefully consider all the choices, including medications or even surgery, tailored to their individual risk. The book, however, has won over thousands of women around the world, from South Africa and Australia to England, Ireland, and Germany.

But the book also won over another convert — me. It may sound silly, but I soon found myself eating the Breast Cancer Prevention Diet. Sure, I wanted to be supportive in my wife's effort to prevent cancer, but I couldn't have been more amazed by the rewards. Within a month, I was 10 pounds lighter and requiring 60 minutes less sleep each night. My workouts were longer and harder. I was more alert and focused at work. My mood had brightened.

You might say, "Hey, you're a guy. You can't get breast cancer." You're right — only about 1 percent of all breast cancer is diagnosed in men. But men do get another cancer . . . prostate cancer. And the more you learn about prostate cancer, the more you'll see amazing similarities. Breast and prostate cancer are even called brother-and-sister cancers. For instance, comparable numbers of men and women get and die from prostate and breast cancer each year . . . with diagnosis rates higher for prostate cancer and death rates higher for breast cancer. In 1996, for example, 24.3 American women per 100,000 died of breast cancer, and 24.1 American men per 100,000 died of prostate cancer; and 110.7 women per 100,000 were diagnosed with breast cancer, while 135.7 men per 100,000 were diagnosed with prostate cancer.[1] The American Cancer Society estimates that for 1999, around 179,300 new cases of prostate cancer were diagnosed and 37,000 men died of the disease, while 176,300 new cases of breast cancer were diagnosed, with 43,700 women dying of the disease. For both cancers, a family history of the disease increases your risk. Both are cancers driven by the body's sex hormones. And both are strongly related to nutrition. In fact, most of the foods that influence breast cancer growth and development also influence the growth and development of prostate cancer.

I called my friend Dr. Dean Ornish and asked him if a breast cancer prevention diet could help protect me against prostate cancer. He invited me to have dinner with him and his lovely wife, Molly, in San Francisco. We had a stunning meal at the wonderful Fleur de Lys Restaurant . . . eating foods containing vanishingly little fat but bursting with great taste and delivering an hours-long food "high." Dean said:

> I think we're at a place with respect to prostate cancer and breast cancer very similar to where we were with respect to coronary heart disease twenty-three years ago when I began conducting research. At that time, there was evidence from animal studies, epidemiological research, and anecdotal case reports in humans indicating that the progression of coronary heart disease might be affected by making comprehensive changes in diet and lifestyle, but no one had conducted a randomized controlled trial to find out. Over time, my colleagues and I at the nonprofit Preventive Medicine Research Institute demonstrated that heart disease often can be slowed, stopped, or even reversed when people make much bigger changes in diet and lifestyle than had previously been recommended. It is possible that we may be at a similar place with respect to early prostate cancer, breast cancer, and perhaps colon cancer.

Dean is directing the first randomized controlled trial in collaboration with Dr. Peter Carroll at UCSF and Dr. William Fair at Memorial Sloan-Kettering Cancer Center to see whether or not the progression of early prostate cancer may be affected by a similar type of lifestyle program that Dr. Ornish found could often reverse coronary heart disease. Says Dean: "Whatever we show will be of great interest. If we show that it affects prostate cancer, then this may give many people new choices. But even if we find it doesn't, then people need to know that as well."

For a *Dateline NBC* program on prostate cancer, I interviewed a man in Dr. Ornish's study. He had embraced Dr. Ornish's lifestyle regimen to combat the disease, including diet, exercise, group support, and stress reduction. He showed me a sophisticated scan, called an MRI spectroscopy scan, of his cancer before he started the program and one from a year or so later. The second scan showed reduced tumor activity. His tumor activity appeared to have declined along with his PSA. Dr. Ornish warned me that this was just the case of a single individual; the scan might not be accurate and was not final proof that lifestyle alone worked as a method of treating prostate cancer.

But I thought, Gee, if the diet-and-lifestyle program showed that much potential in men who already have cancer, what would it do to men like me who just want to prevent it? Wouldn't it have an even more powerful effect? I talked with Mike Milken, founder of CaP CURE (the Association for the Cure of Cancer of the Prostate), an organization dedicated to the cure of prostate cancer. He was among the first to champion nutrition as a way of protecting yourself against prostate cancer. He personally funded much of the important research in the field. He has even published two hugely successful recipe books, *The Taste for Living Cookbook* and *The Taste for Living WORLD Cookbook,* for men trying to protect themselves from prostate cancer and for men who already have the dreaded disease. The recipes demonstrate that you can satisfy your palate at the same time that you're protecting your health. Mike and chef Beth Ginsberg even figured out how to prepare a Reuben sandwich that is prostate healthy! What I saw unfolding was a great untold secret: nutrition is emerging as one of the most important ways of protecting yourself against prostate cancer.

My dinner with Dean and talk with Mike gave me the courage and conviction to commit myself fully to a diet to protect myself against prostate cancer. It's one of the best decisions I've ever made and one I hope to share with you. Sure, not every last piece of research is in. Some would even say it's early in the game. But men of action are used to making bold decisions based on incomplete data. Men buy companies, run political campaigns, wage wars, invent new products, start new companies, research new therapies, all based on the best available — but incomplete — data. In medicine, there's even a term for the method used to take available data and make a firm decision. It's called "evidence-based medicine," as reported in the *Journal of the American Medical Association,* and involves "integrating current best evidence." For nutrition I call it evidence-based nutritional therapy. This is a method of taking all the available nutritional evidence — from test tubes, animal studies, human studies, you name it — and formulating a plan of action. Sure, you could wait twenty years for the research to be completed, but why wait? My own personal belief and that of many researchers is that prostate cancer is just one of a package of diseases that we put ourselves at risk for by consuming what nutritionists call the "Western diet," characterized by high amounts of animal fats, refined flours and sugars, and appallingly small amounts of fiber and whole foods such as fruits, vegetables, whole grains, and cereals. That package of diseases includes diabetes, obesity, heart disease, and, yes, cancer. Around the planet, societies are adopting the Western diet . . . and the

Western diet is leaving millions of victims in its wake, like a great, worldwide scourge. From Southeast Asia to East Africa to the deserts of the American Southwest, heart disease and diabetes are reaching record levels in traditional societies that have made the switch to Western foods. Look for yourself at the handwriting on the wall. The epidemic levels of obesity in America are driven by too much of the wrong kinds of foods. In less than a decade, the number of overweight Americans has climbed by an astonishing 50 percent. In America and around the world there is a new diabetes epidemic, with the number of cases tripling since the 1950s.

While we're far from having the final answers on prostate cancer, the lifestyle presented in this book is very important to your overall longevity and your ability to protect yourself against the ravages of the leading killers in America, from heart disease and diabetes to several important cancers. The Surgeon General's office claims that four of the ten leading causes of death are associated with dietary factors — coronary heart disease, some kinds of cancer, stroke, and Type II diabetes. These health conditions are estimated to cost society over $200 billion each year in medical expenses and lost productivity. The National Cancer Institute links a third of all cancers to the foods that we eat.

Now let's look at prostate cancer itself. Here's a brief primer: The prostate is the shape of a walnut and surrounds the beginning of the *urethra*. Found at the center of the penis, the urethra is the narrow tube that carries urine from the bladder. The prostate gland is composed of hundreds of tiny *glands* which are surrounded and supported by fibrous and muscular *tissue*. These glands manufacture a milky white fluid that is secreted during ejaculation and is a part of semen. The gland is surrounded by a capsule. Theoretically, you could do perfectly well without a prostate after fathering your children. That's because the prostate gland is not required to maintain an erection or achieve orgasm.

Prostate cancer is the malignant transformation and growth of cells in the prostate. Usually the cancer starts in the main glandular part of the prostate. The cancer may spread outside the prostate by extending through the capsule. It may spread locally to lymph nodes or seminal vesicles or it may spread well beyond the prostate, with bone being the most common site for metastasis.

Years ago, the latent, "undiagnosed" form of prostate cancer was often thought of as an incidental finding at autopsy in very old men. In medical school we were told this is a form of cancer you more often die with, not a cancer you die from. Now a remarkable new study by Wael Sakr, M.D., associate professor at Wayne State University in Detroit, and Gabriel Haas, M.D., professor of urology at the State University of New York in Syracuse, shows that the numbers of much younger men with latent cancer as an incidental finding at autopsy are far larger than anyone had imagined.

Until recently it was generally accepted that only a third of men over age 50 harbored what is termed a latent prostate cancer — in other words, a cancer that does not appear, at the time it is inspected, to be a threat to the life or well-being of those who have it. In essence, a latent cancer lies dormant and could remain so throughout your lifetime. But those older studies had two shortcomings. First, not the entire prostate gland was examined. Second, subjects were selected from hospitalized patients and so tended to be older and sicker, and few studies took into consideration younger men or large numbers of African Americans.

Dr. Sakr and his colleagues collaborated with the Wayne

County medical examiner's office to include a thorough microscopic examination of the prostate as part of the regular autopsy procedure for men dying as young as age 20 from accidents and trauma. Dr. Sakr evaluated over 600 prostate glands in a period of four years. He examined samples within a short time of the estimated time of death. All researchers knew about the subjects was their age and race.

The percentages of men with latent prostate cancers were staggering:

- 25% of men in their 30s
- 30% of men in their 40s
- 40% of men in their 50s
- 50–60% of men in their 60s
- 70% of men in their 70s

Should those latent cancers waken from their dormant state and become clinical cancer, the consequences could be disastrous. The bottom line: nearly half of us have these latent cancers as we enter middle age, while the majority of us have them by the time we enter old age. These latent cancers are a wild card. In some men, they will remain quiescent. In others they may grow into a clinically significant tumor. In still others they may grow quickly, even ferociously. The greatest danger is when clinical prostate cancer occurs early in life. Early-onset clinical prostate cancer is a serious disease with high mortality, since younger patients are likely to have more-aggressive tumors that have broken through the capsule of the prostate and metastasized to other parts of the body.

Clinical prostate cancer, even when caught early and treated, stands out as strikingly different from most cancers because of its potentially destructive effect on the way we live. You can recover from early-stage colon cancer or certain skin cancers, for example, without any noticeable effect on your lifestyle. But prostate cancer threatens the very essence of being a male. Here's why. Surgical removal of the prostate is the main curative treatment for prostate cancer. Even though the prostate is a small organ, it's very tough for surgeons to get at. The operation is long and arduous. The recovery can take months. But here's the bad news. There can be major side effects of surgery, even for small, early-stage tumors. You may very nicely survive the operation — or even be cured — only to live for decades with the two main complications: incontinence and impotence. Fortunately, at least half of the men operated on will escape those longer-term complications. With a special new surgery, described later in this book, even fewer men may suffer long-term complications. Still, most men suffer some temporary impotence or incontinence that can last months. Radiation therapy and radioactive seed implants are alternative therapies, but these also have side effects such as incontinence, bowel irritability, and sexual dysfunction.

A prostate cancer outcomes study, published in the January 2000 issue of the *Journal of the American Medical Association* (*JAMA*), found that 18 or more months following radical prostatectomy, 8.4 percent of men were still incontinent and a whopping 59.9 percent were still impotent.

I've called this book *The Prostate Cancer Protection Plan* for a good reason. No one knows how latent prostate cancers start. At present, there is no known way to prevent that latent cancer from starting. In many of us the cancer lies dormant for decades. However, something causes the dormant cancer to spring to life and become a clinically significant cancer. For most men, I'll argue in the next chapter, that something is diet. I've written this book to help you protect yourself against this fateful transition from latent disease to life-threatening cancer. Little realized is just how awful death from prostate cancer is. Michael Korda describes it well in his superb personal account, *Man to Man:* "The only two people I knew closely who had it [prostate cancer] died of it, descending by small agonizing steps into a world of such pain and suffering that those who loved them prayed only for their death."[2] Men by their very nature have historically believed in protecting themselves. But with prostate cancer, for many of us, including me, the natural reaction is to say: "Naw . . . , not me." The surprising truth, as we've just seen from Dr. Sakr's study, is that it is not unlikely that you *do* have a microscopic prostate cancer at this very moment, one that in most cases is lying dormant. Even if there's little you can do to prevent it from forming, there's lots you can do to protect yourself against that latent cancer growing to harm you. That's why this book is called *The Prostate Cancer Protection Plan* — it's a guide to protecting yourself against the cancer that may already be growing within you.

Since much of this protection program relies on lifestyle changes, you might ask why on earth any sensible person would change so much of his lifestyle to beat *one* disease. That is, why not choose instead a program of prevention for colon cancer, heart disease, or stroke? Why just prostate cancer? As we've just seen, prostate cancer is unique in its ability to destroy your quality of life. The other reason to focus so intently on prostate cancer is this. The combined measures that you can undertake to protect yourself against prostate cancer are the same nutritional measures you would use to prevent heart disease, stroke, obesity, diabetes, and colon and other cancers. In fact, heart disease serves as a remarkable sentinel for your risk of prostate cancer. The higher your risk of coronary artery disease, the higher your risk of prostate cancer! A study from the Columbia College of Physicians and Surgeons states it clearly: "Patients with coronary heart disease may represent a high-risk group for prostate cancer."[3] Why? The same grand and excessive lifestyle and diet that lead you down the road to heart disease may also lead you down the road to prostate cancer, and vice versa. Heart disease has long been the greatest fear of men in the prime of their lives. But with advances in the treatment and prevention of heart disease, that fear is quickly being replaced by dread of prostate cancer.

What's laid out in this book is not, however, a general program. The measures are highly specific and targeted toward prostate cancer, but the benefits spread across the vast majority of health risks that you face.

Twenty years ago, prostate cancer research was considered by some to be a medical backwater with few researchers, fewer effective research tools, and a staggering percentage of men who presented to their doctors an advanced, lethal cancer. Thanks to visionaries such as Dr. William Catalano, Dr. Patrick Walsh, and Mike Milken, and institutions such as CaP CURE and the National Cancer Institute, there is a bright new future for men with the disease. Early aggressive screening and treatment may already be decreasing deaths from prostate cancer. Other visionaries, for example Dr. Dean Ornish, forecast that early prostate cancer may be a more dynamic cancer, whose course may be changed, perhaps even reversed, far more quickly than we ever believed. Most alluring is research seeking to transform prostate cancer into a chronic disease that may be treated very much like high blood pressure or high cholesterol — in other words, treated *before* a catastrophic event occurs. With the right protection plan, you can track and stalk this cancer before it becomes big enough to haunt you.

For those of you who already have prostate cancer, here's what Mike Milken, the founder of CaP CURE, has to say: "First, cancer is not a death sentence. Second, you as an individual can play a huge role in your own cancer. You have to have a positive attitude and be aggressive. Changing your diet and exercising are things you can do to increase the *quality* and possibly the *quantity* of your life."

Special Note to Women

There's an extraordinary reason why women should be concerned about prostate cancer in the men they love and men about breast cancer in the women they love. As we've seen, breast cancer and prostate cancer are very much brother-and-sister diseases. Researchers have found a correlation between the breast cancer gene BRCA2 and prostate cancer.[4] A family history of breast cancer seems to increase chances of fatal prostate cancer. Even in the absence of a family history of prostate cancer, men with a family history of breast cancer "showed a modest increased risk of fatal prostate cancer."[5] So if you do have a family history of breast cancer, you'll want to consider the added risk your father, brothers, or sons may have of possibly fatal prostate cancer.

But it's not just genes; environment also seems to count. One study showed that prostate and breast cancer are more frequent in married couples than in the general population. In other words, in a marriage in which a wife develops breast cancer, the man is more likely to develop prostate cancer. And when the husband has developed prostate cancer, the wife is more likely to develop breast cancer. "A combination of carcinoma of the prostate and female breast sites was found in 18 couples versus 5.4 expected in the general population," one study reports.[6] The most logical explanation is that the married man and woman share a common environment. At the top of that environment is food.

So what can you do? Both cancers, research shows, are highly dependent on *food as fuel*. So when husbands and wives share the same diet, they may share a cancer risk. To the extent that a woman limits her own risk of breast cancer with changes in diet, she limits the prostate cancer risk for the man or men she lives with — husbands, sons, and fathers. You will find that the prostate cancer protection diet mirrors a breast cancer prevention diet. That is fortunate, because it means that husbands and wives, sons and daughters, can eat the same foods to prevent different cancers. Start today with the shared goal of protecting yourselves against cancer with a shared diet.

While prostate and breast cancer are brother-and-sister diseases, prostate cancer is a poor younger brother to breast cancer. Women have done an amazing job of organizing themselves to push for more research, for greater awareness, and to emphasize the early screening that can catch cancer before it becomes a lethal disease. We men have been less aware of the disease and its impact. We've been late to organize and to push for the science we so desperately need. We've learned a great deal, but we still have a great deal more to learn from the example women have set in their remarkable fight against breast cancer.

The Road Map

This book is very straightforward. **Part I** presents the most compelling arguments there are that prostate cancer is a nutritional disease. We'll learn the lessons of men in other countries who have strikingly less prostate cancer than we do here in the United States.

Part II gives you all of the treasured foods that can protect you against this killer. Each food has strong scientific validation. For men tired of hearing, "Just eat more fruits and vegetables," you'll find fun and exciting foods that come with solid scientific backing. I've long believed that foods are the most powerful preventive medicines there are. In fact, the most fascinating part of this book is reading about the highly targeted drug-like effect that so many foods have. At the end of each of these chapters, you'll find a section called What You Can Do Now. Until another decade or so has passed, it's unlikely that you'll find formal recommendations; for that reason, I've included this section to lay out what the safest, most effective, and most reasonable course of action is until the final results are in.

There is the enticing idea that many of the foods found in Part II could be combined into a single program, as part of a larger, lifestyle change. This is discussed in Part III. Just as doctors attack a certain clinical cancer in a variety of ways, with combinations of chemotherapy, radiation, and surgery, why not try to stop a latent cancer from growing by attacking it in different and powerful ways?

Clearly, the best plan involves using many protective agents that are low in risk but act in strikingly different ways — in a word, that way is diet. Part III draws together the smorgasbord of protective foods from Part II into the balanced diet you'll want for your own prostate cancer protection program. You'll find actual meal plans. For those of us who live life on the road, you'll also find a guide to eating out and eating on the run with foods that are both fast and spectacularly healthy. However, first and foremost you'll find cuisines known to be associated with astonishingly low rates of prostate cancer in other countries. These specific cuisines are the best way of including the most important elements from Part II. Why? To incorporate so many different foods into your diet, you'll want a cuisine that has stood the test of time. Rather than a tasteless assortment of superfoods, you'll find terrific meals that deliver fabulous taste and tremendous energy. That's because they've been developed over thousands of years by populations who treasure these foods for the good health and the enjoyment of life they deliver. They've stood the test of time.

Rounding out a prostate-healthy lifestyle are stress-busting and fitness plans. I've included a chapter on each, in order to give you every possible protective measure that has strong backing. As time passes, researchers may prove some of these measures more powerful than others. It's possible that in five or so years, a protection plan might have fewer elements. The strategy here is including all possible measures so you won't miss anything that could be beneficial. That may result in a little overkill, but since each of these measures is part of a vigorous, healthy life, the only side effect is that you'll be that much healthier!

Part IV includes the other key ways of protecting yourself — medications, supplements, surgery, and an important blood test that can serve as your early warning system. This test may play an even more important role in your future, that is, warning you *before* you get into trouble so you can take action through the steps outlined in this book. We are entering a new and exciting era. The old paradigm was that of early diagnosis and early treatment. The new paradigm is that of early detection and prevention.

Part V presents the real programs of men protecting themselves against prostate cancer and men who already have the disease and are fighting it. Many of them ingeniously incorporate all the steps in this book into their own personal regimens. I've learned a lot from them and hope you will as well.

The **Appendices** contain a special chapter on evaluating your risk of prostate cancer for your given age, race, and family history. There is also a more detailed scientific discussion of some important elements in the book. To be frank, this is a highly technical area filled with nearly impenetrable scientific concepts. This book is written for the lay reader, not for research scientists. While the main body of the book presents the most important arguments, it tries to avoid getting lost in the excruciating detail of research studies. I'll admit to doing a double take as I plowed through some of the thousands of papers already published in this field — pretty dense stuff. The Appendices, however, do draw the research out in greater detail for those of you who want to read further.

Since there is growing consumer anger about the confusing messages in the media about nutrition, I've tried to make each recommendation as clear as possible and to leave the debate for the Appendices. If it's healthy and good for you in general, and has a credible beneficial effect on the prostate, you'll find it here. This book includes every reasonable measure to protect yourself against prostate cancer so that you give yourself the best opportunity of staying well. Each of these measures is safe and part of a rigorous, healthy lifestyle. Says Dr. Ornish: "This program improves your quality of life, not just your survival, and not years later but a week or two later. When you make big changes you get big benefits. These big benefits reframe the reason for changing diet and lifestyle from fear of dying to joy of living . . . and that's what ultimately helps people sustain the program."

Prostate cancer was long dismissed as a disease of old age. Implied in that is that it doesn't matter if you get prostate cancer if you are "old." My grandfather lived to the age of 91. He didn't die with prostate cancer, he died of it. You may say, Gee, 91, pretty good. But if you were to have met my grandfather at age 90, you would have met an energetic man who looked and acted 60. He enjoyed every minute of his vigorous life. Life was no less important or dear to him at 90 than it was at 50. My brothers, sisters, and I loved every minute we were with him. We treasured his stories, his jokes, his kindness, and his wonderful spirit. More and more of us are going to live decades longer than we ever imagined and in great good health. But whether you are 45 or 95, when prostate cancer strikes, it brings with it a terrible price in terms of discomfort, pain, and theft of your quality of life. Prostate cancer in young men certainly gets our attention. It's unnerving and even frightening. But the majority of us won't get prostate cancer when we're young, we'll get it as we age. Even if you're not at risk of prostate cancer as a young man, it is a disease you will want to make every effort to protect yourself against. The risk increases dramatically with each passing decade. The earlier you start to protect yourself, the better. Today we're a youth-oriented culture that too often dismisses people simply because they're "old," but I'll never forget the words of UCLA heart transplant surgeon Dr. Hillel Laks. When I asked him about the value of saving older patients using transplant surgery, he looked at me and simply said: "Every life is infinitely precious." Our grandfather's certainly was to us.

Part One

A Nutritional Disease

Men in Japan and China have up to 90 percent less prostate cancer than American men. That's an astounding statistic. Ninety percent! Most men I talk to are at first surprised at the huge disparity. Their second reaction is to sort of shrug and say, "It's in the genes, nothing much you can do about that." But that's where they're wrong. The best evidence points squarely to a difference in nutrition as a much bigger major factor. The evidence is fascinating. Laurence Kolonel, M.D., Ph.D., professor at the University of Hawaii, hit on a brilliant research strategy. Why not study men who migrated from the Far East to the United States and see if their risk of cancer increased? After all, emigrating wouldn't change their genetic makeup. What happened? Bingo! Dr. Kolonel hit the nail on the head. "I would say that the case of migrants is the strongest indication that the environment is influencing prostate cancer risk," he says. He showed that when the Japanese move away from Japan, their rates of prostate cancer *do* increase. Now most "migrant studies," as they are called, show the greatest increased risk in the children and grandchildren of the migrants. And that's what you'd expect. The first generation would largely maintain their traditional ways, and the younger generations would adapt more readily to the new environment: burgers, fries, pizza, sodas, drive-ins, video games . . . you name it! That's precisely what happens with breast cancer rates. Asian women living in Asia have 90 percent less breast cancer than American women. But when Asian women move to America, it's their daughters and granddaughters whose rates of breast cancer close in on those of American women. What's so striking about Dr. Kolonel's studies is this. For men who moved from Japan to Hawaii, Dr. Kolonel found a *large* increase in prostate cancer rates in the migrants themselves! Say a man emigrates from Japan to Hawaii at age twenty: by the age of fifty, his risk of a clinically significant prostate cancer is much higher than it would have been had he stayed in Japan! Dr. Kolonel found that the risk doubled in these migrants. Here's what he concluded: "Migrants have the same genetic makeup as their families back home, and so it must be something external that is causing the risk change." So, if environment is changing risk, the question becomes *what* in the environment is affecting risk? Which lifestyle component is raising risk? Suggests Dr. Kolonel: "Diet is a good candidate. When Japanese migrants come to Hawaii, the biggest area of change for them is diet since Hawaii is not a heavily industrialized or polluted state. What changes here is exposure to Western diet."

What is this Western diet? Dr. Kolonel explains that it's a diet heavily based on animal products — particularly meat and dairy products — and therefore higher in fat, especially animal fat, than the diet of more traditional populations in Asia and Africa. As populations become more Westernized, they shift away from whole grains and cereals toward meat and dairy, and this changes the nature of their fat intake to more saturated fats. In comparison to the diets of Africa and Asia, the Western diet contains a lower intake of fruits and vegetables.

Now let's take a closer look at prostate cancer numbers. We read in the introduction that many of us have a latent cancer, even at a fairly young age. You'll recall that even for men in their 30s, 25 percent have latent cancer. Here's the big surprise. Latent cancer is not unique to the United States. Researchers find that, at any given age, men all over the world share the same risk for latent cancers. They have the same percentage of latent cancers at the same ages we do. You might be tempted to say: Huh? I thought you said men in other countries, especially the Far East, have less cancer. Well I did. They have less *clinical* cancer, but not less latent cancer.

Remember, latent cancer is in a quiescent stage that poses no harm. Let's take China as an example. Chinese men have the same percentage of latent cancer as American men. That's right. They have just as much latent cancer as you or I. But hold on! How many of those latent cancers become a clinically important cancer? In China, the answer is extremely few. Clinical rates in China are the lowest in the world at 2.8 per 100,000 people a year. American whites have 100 per 100,000. That's *thirty-six* times higher than rates in China. So if American and Chinese men start at square one with the same amount of latent cancer, what accounts for the difference in rates of clinical cancer? Why do these latent cancers spring to life in so many American men and not in Chinese men? What is the fuel that transforms a benign, latent tumor into a life-threatening one? In a word, diet. Charles Myers, M.D., of the University of Virginia, also concludes: "Diet definitely affects the progression of prostate cancer from a microscopic level to a metastatic level."

Here's the real irony. Sure, men eating traditional foods in the Far East have low rates of cancer, but what about those men tempted by a change to a Western diet? When they do switch, watch out. Take the burgeoning metropolis of Shanghai, where it's becoming as easy to get a burger, fries, and a shake as it is to get spring rolls and tofu. The rate of clinical prostate cancer is now beginning to rise among those men who have crossed the line from traditional to Western foods. Ann Hsing, Ph.D., epidemiologist at the National Cancer Institute, conducted a study in Shanghai to examine why prostate cancer rates were increasing. She analyzed the diets of men at high risk for prostate cancer. Sure enough. What were they eating? For starters, more animal fats, especially red meat, and preserved foods such as preserved meats and vegetables. With increased animal product intake, more calories were coming from animal fat. Add to that lots more calories than the Chinese traditionally eat. The result: these men weren't just getting prostate cancer, they were also fat. In fact, they developed the most dangerous kind of obesity, called central obesity, which occurs when fat piles up around your midsection. Central obesity is commonly seen in people who eat large amounts of starches, refined flours, and sugars. The good news is that the men who ate healthier traditional foods and vegetables such as garlic, scallions, and onions had a lower risk. The traditional Chinese diet has more fiber, plenty of fruits, and lots of soybeans, green leafy vegetables, and orange vegetables such as pumpkin. In the traditional Chinese diet, 60 percent of energy intake came from complex carbohydrates. "I think our findings corroborate findings in the U.S.," says Dr. Hsing.

How Big a Villain Is the Western Diet?

The Japanese flat-out blame the Western diet for their prostate cancer travails: There were 5,399 deaths from prostate cancer in 1995 in Japan. By 2015 that number will increase to 13,494. Dr. Y. Kakehi of the Department of Urology, Faculty of Medicine, Kyoto University, concludes: "Change in dietary habit (more Western-style diet) is considered to be a major cause of the increase."

English researchers too have concluded that nutrition is the major risk factor associated with prostate cancer, singling out low intake of fresh fruit, low intake of vegetables, and low intake of whole-grain cereal, as well as excess body fat.[1]

The Association for the Cure of Cancer of the Prostate (CaP CURE) writes in its white paper on nutrition: "Of all the risk factors for prostate cancer, only nutrition seems to explain the differences in global distribution of this disease."[2] Studies estimate that 75 percent of all cases of prostate cancer could be prevented by changes in diet and lifestyle. Scientists from Cap CURE conclude: "We believe, therefore, that nutrition and lifestyle practices in lower-risk countries arrest the growth of prostate cancer so that it is never clinically discovered."[3]

Okay, you may say, what does all of this high-powered epidemiologic research have to do with me? After reading the thorough research on nutrition and prostate cancer, I have to tell you that I'm convinced. As a physician and as a male concerned about prostate cancer, I believe this research is the strongest indication that diet plays a big role in prostate cancer and that there is something you can do about your own diet to change your risk. This isn't just a pipe dream; this could be close to the whole game. But I asked myself: Which foods? What diet? Well, you're in for a real treat. There is a true treasure trove of terrific foods that can help protect you against prostate cancer. If you're like me, you don't just want to read a lot of wishful thinking by well-meaning advocates of alternative medicine. You want hard facts. The hard facts, in this case, show that foods have highly specific effects on the prostate gland. These are varied enough to give you a range of strategies to protect yourself. You'll also find, as I have, that this is high-level science. Foods have incredibly sophisticated powers, like well-designed pharmaceuticals. Researchers are excited enough about the power of foods that they're already intensely investigating many of them. In fact, tens of millions of dollars are being spent on nutritional research. The next section of the book will present these foods and tease apart their specific actions that can help you protect yourself against prostate cancer. You'll be pleased to learn that virtually all of them have terrific general health benefits, from lowering your cholesterol and your risk of heart disease to controlling your weight and risk of other cancers. They are also foods that will make you feel terrific, perhaps the best you have ever felt. I hope you'll develop the same enthusiasm for the foods and meals in this book that I have. Tens of thousands of men threatened with prostate cancer have already made the change. Most telling of all, men who already have the disease are finding remarkable changes in the state of their cancer with a rigorous change in diet.

Why? The most intriguing reason is that our bodies are designed to eat a specific diet. Just as putting low-grade, cheap gas into a car will eventually ruin a car engine, putting cheap fuels that we were not designed to use into our own bodies will lead to disease. Specifically, the human prostate and the Western diet may be incompatible. You see, through human evolution, our bodies became accustomed to specific foods. Unfortunately, our bodies can't turn on a dime and acclimatize overnight to a new diet, especially one loaded with animal fats and refined carbohydrates, almost devoid of fruits and vegetables. Human evolution marks time in the tens of thousands of years. The dramatic changes in our diets since the Industrial Revolution aren't even a tick on our evolutionary clocks. What's the diet we as men are meant to eat? Is it roast beef with Yorkshire pudding, roasted potatoes, and gravy? Not if you look back into the dawn of humankind.

For 90 percent of the last 200,000 years, we were fruit-and-vegetable eaters. Donald Coffey, Ph.D., who is a professor in the famed Department of Urology at Johns Hopkins, argues that humankind did not evolve fully equipped to be dairy or meat eaters. More to the point, our prostates may not have evolved to handle a diet rich in fats. Humans came from an arm of evolution that did not eat a lot of meat. Until 2.5 million years ago, we were mainly gatherers — we ate seeds and fruits and nuts. Homo sapiens first appeared 100,000 years ago, but only 9,000 years ago did we start processing and storing food and trading it. That's when we started down the road to eating the massive amounts of carbohydrates that we eat today, for example, corn, wheat, rice, barley, potatoes, and root plants. Fruit consumption dropped, since fruits were harder to store. And as we increasingly ate a diet rich in meat, which we cooked and even burned, we stopped eating as many fruits and vegetables. Dairy got big only around 3,000 years ago, and it's then that we increased our dairy intake. Before that we would get milk from goats and sheep, but it was only when we bred these animals that we developed the dairy industry.

"After fifty years of trying to prevent cancer, we've learned that we should go back to eating the foods we ate while we were evolving," says Dr. Coffey. He adds, "It's not surprising that the American Cancer Society and the National Cancer Institute make the same suggestions. They tell us to return to the diet we ate when we were evolving: more vegetables, more fruit, more fiber, less red meat, less animal fat, less dairy, less barbecuing, and more aerobic exercise." So who eats a diet closer to the one we were designed to eat? In parts of China, people eat around 6 to 8 percent fat. Compare that to the United States, where the figure is 30 to 40 percent, much of it animal fat. "Put it all together and you'll figure that our lifestyle is giving us cancer," says Dr. Coffey. I swear the reason I feel so terrific on this diet is that it's the one we're supposed to eat, the one we are designed to eat.

The great good news is that there *is* a diet that humans were designed to eat and a diet that can be highly protective against prostate cancer. The evidence is so strong that many top physicians in the best academic centers put their patients on a "prostate cancer diet." But don't take my word for it; just look at what the top experts have to say about diet in their own patients with prostate cancer.

- Charles Myers, M.D., of UVA, says: "I recommend a diet change as an adjunct to treatment to every patient. I don't recommend a diet change as a sole treatment. However, some men have very slow-growing cancers — their tumors double every four to five years. In that subset a change in diet may be enough." Dr. Myers recommends essentially the same diet that Milken and Ornish recommend.
- Erik Goluboff, M.D., of Columbia University, says: "I put all of my patients on a prostate cancer diet."

I'm impressed that so many experts believe that diet could have an effect even on men who already have prostate cancer. Even more compelling than the use of a prostate cancer diet in treatment of patients is the growing interest in a prostate cancer diet for prevention.

- "Even if you're dealt a bad hand in terms of your prostate cancer genetics, such as faulty male sex hormone receptors, diet may still influence the likelihood of that cancer turning bad," says Christopher Logothetis, M.D., of M. D. Anderson Cancer Center at the University of Texas in Houston.

- "Diet will hinder or help mutations that could lead to the development of a tumor," says Linda Nebeling, Ph.D., M.P.H., R.D., nutritionist at the National Cancer Institute.

What about real patients on the front lines of this disease? Bob Each is a survivor of late-stage prostate cancer, and he says: "For me, it's a race. I've got to run long enough to get to the cure. The diet is one way to keep me running. The diet helps keep me stay focused on suppressing the disease."

Dean Ornish, M.D., is America's foremost expert on nutrition and disease prevention. More than two decades ago he began his quest to prove that heart disease could be reversed with a stringent lifestyle program. He succeeded by showing that blockages in coronary arteries actually became smaller. The arteries opened up as symptoms dramatically improved. So successful is the program that many major insurers now pay for this "alternative" means of treating heart disease. Medicare is now conducting a demonstration project of Dr. Ornish's program for reversing heart disease in sites around the country.

Now Dr. Ornish and his colleagues are targeting prostate cancer. They have carefully designed for men with prostate cancer a program consisting of a rigorous diet, meditation, group support, and exercise. Their intent is to determine if this experimental program may slow or even stop the progression of cancer. The men studied all have biopsy-proven cancer. Dr. Ornish cautions that the results he has to date are not final and that the trial is far from over. There are, however, some intriguing trends. In Dr. Ornish's heart disease reversal program and in his weight control program, the more carefully men adhered to the program, the better they did. This may end up being true of the prostate study as well. I urge you to follow carefully the results as they appear in the media and in professional journals.

What is the proof Dr. Ornish and others are looking for? The bottom line is, does the program save lives? That's the gold standard that hard-nosed researchers are looking for. Until results are in, there are what are called intermediate markers. These are objective scientific measures of real progress, and they're quite valuable. One reason is that there is a great sense of reward when you can see real results. You know you're moving in the right direction. Markers tell researchers that they are changing what they want to change. Since prostate cancer can take decades to develop, it could be many years before you know if you've succeeded in protecting yourself against the disease. The same is true with other diseases. Take heart disease as an example. Doctors and patients rely on intermediate markers, the most well known of which is the cholesterol test. Patients take great satisfaction in lowering their cholesterol levels, although it does not guarantee that they will avoid a heart attack.

As foods are increasingly put to the test in the lab and in clinical trials, more and more doctors are beginning to view diet as *nutritional therapy*. Dr. Ernst Wynder, the late founder of the American Health Foundation, pioneered the term *nutritional therapy*, that is, using specific foods to treat an actual illness or prevent a latent one from becoming full blown. Researchers use for foods the words *chemoprevention* and *chemoprotection*. What's the difference between prevention and protection? Prevention is avoiding foods or substances that might cause cancer — for example, high-fat foods. Protection is taking foods or substances, such as lycopene or soy, that may actively protect you against a potentially cancerous process in your body. You'll find both of these strategies used in this book.

Many men look somewhat askance at the idea of foods as therapy, perhaps believing that I mean foods work through some kind of mystical force. Foods don't work through magic; they work like drugs, with highly specific effects on receptors, cells, enzymes, and biochemical pathways throughout the body. We'll look at these specific effects of the active ingredients found in foods: for instance, lycopene, found in tomatoes, sulforaphane, found in broccoli, and genistein, found in soy foods. Studies are showing that some foods may protect you against a cancer growing in the first place — an example is antioxidants, which may cut down on damage done to genetic material. Some strategies, such as soy protein intake, may slow or stop a microscopic tumor from becoming an important clinical case of prostate cancer. Other strategies, such as decreasing animal fat intake, may decrease the risk of metastasis, while still others could help prevent a recurrence.

The foods, drugs, and supplements discussed in this book are primarily for men who'd like to protect themselves against developing a clinical cancer. However, many of these approaches are also used by men who already have prostate cancer. In fact fully 30 percent of prostate cancer patients use alternative strategies such as nutrition. Some do so in place of any conventional treatment, but most use these methods alongside traditional treatment. If you already have prostate cancer, you'll want to discuss with your doctor what makes the most sense for you. You'll find that urologists are quite up to date on nutritional strategies and often recommend them as part of traditional therapy. Harry Pinchot is a prostate cancer survivor diagnosed with metastatic disease at age 55. He says:

> Diet gives one a sense of empowerment. It gives you a psychological sense of empowerment that you can do something that is an adjunctive therapy to the traditional medical treatment. Proactive patients survive longer than reactive patients. . . . Diet helps maintain hope. It gives you a sense of empowerment that you are doing something to control the disease.

Mike Milken says: "I truly believe that diet can have a preventive effect." As founder and chairman of CaP CURE, he adds: "Our feeling is that with the proper diet you can slow the cancer growth."

Part Two

Foods

Special Note on Commercial Products

Throughout this book you will find commercial product names, Web sites and 800 numbers. These are provided to increase the usefulness of the book and to help you find products that are particularly hard to find or are one of a kind. This does not constitute an endorsement of any of these products either by the author or by organizations named in this book. They are designed to help you overcome the frustration that can often come from trying to find foods, supplements, and information on your own.

Soy

I first met Mike Milken at a radiation therapy center in Los Angeles. After completing an interview for the CBS *Evening News,* we strolled outside. He was clutching what looked like a large coffee can. He carried it as if it were gold. To him it was. Mike was diagnosed with advanced prostate cancer in 1993. Six years later he is disease-free. He wasn't holding a secret, genetically engineered advance formulation. It was soy protein powder. Besides founding the Association for the Cure of Cancer of the Prostate, he has been enormously influential in growing the field of prostate cancer research — he has supported work on nutrition, prevention, and genetic engineering and has promoted clinical trials for advanced disease. Mike has now raised more than $100 million in contributions to CaP CURE in the quest to bring prostate cancer research up by the bootstraps. With all the access he has to the top research centers in the world and to high-tech drugs, I thought he would choose an experimental medication engineered by a top biotech firm. I was stunned that he opted for something as simple and low tech as soy as his protective treatment of choice — soy as part of a healthy low-fat diet like the one recommended by Dr. Dean Ornish and others.

Why soy? Soy is far more than a simple food. Researchers believe that components of soy work as though they were custom-made drug molecules with highly specific actions such as restricting blood vessel growth, blocking receptors in the prostate, and inhibiting critical enzymes.

Of all the different dietary factors that explain the difference in cancer rates between the Far East and the United States, soy may be one of the most important. An extraordinary epidemiological study led by Dr. J. R. Herbert at the University of Massachusetts Medical School looked at 42 countries and tried to correlate international variations in rate of prostate cancer and mortality with diet. In these 42 countries, the effectiveness of soy on a per calorie basis was at least four times as large as that of any other dietary factor, the investigators reported in the *Journal of the National Cancer Institute*[1]; and the more soy men ate, the lower their risk of prostate cancer.

The great irony is that while the U.S. is the largest soy producer in the world, American men eat vanishingly little soy protein. Natives of the Island of Okinawa eat 100 grams a day, and have a small fraction of the cancer we have plus the greatest longevity in the world to boot! In the U.S., however, we eat on average only 3.8 grams a day.

While these observations from other countries give us the greatest hope, studies in the laboratory give us a better sense of how soy works its wonders. Dr. Morris Pollard of the University of Notre Dame found that when he gave soy preparations to animals with a high likelihood of contracting prostate cancer, he could slow the onset of the cancer. And Dr. Donald Coffey of Johns Hopkins, together with Dr. Herman Adlercreutz of Helsinki, Finland, transplanted a human prostate tumor into a rat to examine whether soy would make a difference. They found that in animals soy significantly lowered tumor volume.

Genistein

Although the final verdict on soy and prostate cancer is still out, soy looks like a true wonder food because of its myriad effects. The most powerful component of soy in protecting

Grams of Soy Protein Intake

Country	Grams per Day
U.S.A.	3.8
Taiwan	35
Japan	40
Okinawa	100

you against prostate cancer appears to be genistein. What is genistein? Genistein is secreted in the roots of the soybean. Its role is to attract to the soybean the bacteria that fix nitrogen in the soil. Technically, genistein is a plant estrogen. You needn't be alarmed that you're taking a female hormone, since genistein has only 1/1000th the power of full-strength estrogen. Genistein's real strength is that it acts in nearly a half dozen quite different ways as an anticancer agent. Listed below are the most important mechanisms known to date. Experts emphasize that these different mechanisms don't work independently of one another but are interconnected. The big picture is that genistein can slow cell growth and even the spread of tumors.

Stops New Blood Vessel Growth

Just as an army travels on its stomach, a cancer needs new blood vessels to grow, spread, and metastasize. The tumor's blood supply growth is called angiogenesis. There are two distinct stages of blood vessel growth, or angiogenesis, in prostate cancer development. The first is a "prevascular" phase, in which there is a limited amount of growth but the tumor hasn't completed all the steps necessary to become a full-blown cancer. When the next stage kicks in, there is sub-stantial development of new blood vessels. This finally allows the cancer to grow freely, to spread, and even to metastasize after years of lying in wait. That's why so many preventive medicine experts so strongly favor taking chemoprevention agents that inhibit this blood vessel growth. Dr. Adlercreutz showed that genistein inhibits metastasis by inhibiting the tu-mor's blood vessel growth.

Slows the Prostate Cancer Cell Cycle

The speed at which cells grow and divide is regulated by the speed of the cell cycle. One powerful substance that controls the prostate cancer cell cycle is P-27, which acts as a brake. The more P-27 the better. When P-27 is increased, researchers see a decrease in speed of progression through the cell cycle. Healthy men have an abundance of P-27 in their prostate cells, which keeps the cell cycle in check. Where does genis-tein fit in? Dr. Qingyi Wei of M. D. Anderson found that the intake of genistein increases the P-27 expression. In theory, the more genistein, the more P-27. Steven Hursting, Ph.D., of M. D. Anderson found that genistein, even at fairly low con-centrations, slows down the rate at which the human prostate cancer cells progress through the cell cycle.

Blocks Receptors

Certain compounds signal the cell to increase cell growth. They do so by attaching to receptors that act as on-off switches. Genistein can interfere with the cell signaling by blocking the receptors at two levels. Think of a room with a lighting system that has both a wall switch that if flicked can turn on several lights in the room and a master switch that if off will not permit the wall switch to turn on the lights. Genistein can block both the wall switch and the master switch.

Here's an example of how it can block the wall switch. Epidermal growth factor (EGF) locks onto the receptor in the cell and causes the cell to grow. A group of Japanese researchers led by Dr. T. Akiyama found that genistein is a superb inhibitor of the epidermal growth factor receptor. Genistein blocks the EGF receptor so the cell nucleus does not get this signal to continue growing.

Genistein also blocks the master switch, which Allan Wells, M.D., Ph.D., of the University of Pittsburgh says is the adhesion switch. For the wall switch to work in the first place, the adhesion or stickiness among cells has to be lessened. Responsible for the decrease in stickiness is a class of enzymes called the tyrosine kinases. And genistein blocks the tyrosine kinase receptors so that they can't cause a decrease in stickiness.

Maintains Cell Stickiness

In their normal state cells are tightly linked to other cells. For a cancer to grow, one of the things required is to loosen these adhesions to other cells. In fact, a change in stickiness is one of the differences between tumor cells and normal cells. Cancer cells usually have a decrease in stickiness that allows the cells to grow and travel. Cell migration is important for the cancer growth, because it allows tumor invasion and metastasis. And by blocking the tyrosine-kinase receptors, genistein blocks the tyrosine-kinase pathway that causes less cell stickiness.

Acts As an Antioxidant

Lastly, genistein acts as an antioxidant. Stephen Barnes, Ph.D., and Victor Darley-Usmar, Ph.D., of the University of

Alabama at Birmingham tested the power of genistein against bleach, technically called hypochlorite. Yes, the body makes bleach, which is an important but also potentially harmful oxidant. Hypochlorite is produced in the immune response to kill off invading bacteria, but it doesn't distinguish among the good, the bad, and the ugly — so if it's made chronically, it damages normal tissue. Genistein reacts with hypochlorite and destroys it. This is one way in which genistein acts as an antioxidant, and Dr. Barnes and Dr. Darley-Usmar are now exploring other antioxidant activity of genistein.

Let's take a closer look at what genistein does and how it does it.

- The Strang Cancer Prevention Center in New York City found 100 times higher genistein levels in Japanese men than in Finnish men. Finns eat much the same Western diet we eat. The payoff for the Japanese men was striking. Strang found among the Japanese men only 1/10th the rate of prostate cancer as among the Finns!

- Dr. Sarah Strom of M. D. Anderson Cancer Center undertook a detailed study of 100 men who did have prostate cancer compared to 100 who did not. She found that for the men who did have prostate cancer, their average daily intake of genistein for the year before they were diagnosed was 19.8 micrograms. For those men who didn't have prostate cancer, their average daily intake for the past year was 29.7 micrograms.

- Dr. Barnes found that in culture, genistein inhibited the growth of human prostate cancer cells. Using a relatively large amount of genistein, Dr. Barnes saw a 50 percent reduction in tumor growth. Dr. Barnes's findings were reproduced in several experiments and were found to hold true not only in test tubes but also in animal models.

- Dr. Carol Lamartiniere of the University of Alabama and Dr. Rosemary Schleicher of Emory University studied rats with prostate cancer and showed that by giving the animals genistein they could reduce the numbers of tumors.
- Dr. Jack Geller of the University of California at San Diego took human prostate cancer cells from a man who had had a prostatectomy, examined how adding genistein would affect DNA synthesis, and found that genistein inhibited prostate cancer cell growth. He saw inhibition at ten times less than the amount Dr. Barnes had used in his study demonstrating the awesome potential for genistein in humans.

Key Health Advantages to Soy

At the beginning of this book, I said this diet had changed my life. A big part of the increased energy, alertness, and endurance comes from soy, which might well be considered the ultimate health food. If the cancer research has not convinced you that you should incorporate soy into your diet, the following soy health advantages may.

Lowers Cholesterol

Soy protein is one of the most powerful cholesterol-lowering dietary agents. University of Kentucky's James Anderson, Ph.D., who published in the *New England Journal of Medicine* a now-classic review of soy research, says:

> Our study indicated that consuming 17 to 25 grams of soy protein per day could have meaningful effects on serum cholesterol levels. Soy protein intake was associated with a

9.3 percent reduction in serum cholesterol, a 12.9 percent reduction in serum LDL-cholesterol, and a 10.5 percent reduction in serum triglycerides. HDL-cholesterol [the good kind] levels increased by 2.4 percent.

In October 1999, the Food and Drug Administration (FDA) authorized food producers to include in their labels of foods containing soy protein that it can help reduce the risk of coronary heart disease by reducing cholesterol levels. In order to qualify for the claim, a serving of the food must contain at least 6.25 grams of soy protein (remember that 25 grams of soy protein daily in the diet is needed to show a significant cholesterol-lowering effect).

Great Source of Protein

Soy is 38 percent protein, double the content of many meats. The protein in soy supplies all essential amino acid needs for human health. Soy also has the highest amounts of the amino acid tyrosine, the main building block of neurochemicals that keep you alert. That's why I use it as a terrific waker-upper first thing in the morning.

Protects Bones

Vegetarian women who have higher intakes of soy protein have lower rates of osteoporosis. Several researchers are now studying the use of soy for osteoporosis prevention. Dr. Barnes has studied bone loss prevention in rats and found that adding high levels of genistein (10 to 20 times what the average Asian diet contains) to a standard diet prevented the expected bone loss. Human studies are not conclusive yet, and some researchers would argue that the rate of osteoporosis in Japanese women is the same as in American women but that Japanese women experience fewer hip fractures because their bodies are smaller.

Keeps Blood Sugar Even

Soy was first used to help treat diabetics in 1910! Starches and refined flour and sugar products, on the other hand, can lead to elevated blood sugar levels. Soybeans set the record for slow-burning carbohydrates. Their glycemic index is 15 on a scale that goes to 100. That makes oatmeal, at 49, look like a hot fudge sundae.

Reduces Inflammation

Dr. Herman Adlercreutz found that when he took soy out of the diet of an animal, the animal developed an inflamed prostate, suggesting that soy normally has an anti-inflammatory effect.

Soy Consumer's Guide

Dosage

An authoritative source on nutrition and prostate cancer, Mike Milken's Association for the Cure of Cancer of the Prostate (CaP CURE), recommends that men increase their soy protein intake to 40 grams a day. Most experts agree that there is no harm done at that dose.

In Taiwan, the average dose of soy is 35 grams of soy protein a day taken as foods as part of a normal diet. Starting on page 142, you will find complete meal plans with 40 grams of soy protein a day.

Mike Milken himself consumes over 100 grams of soy each day — two milkshakes a day, each with 40 grams of soy protein, and at least another 20 grams in foods. He told me that this mimics the amount taken by men in Okinawa, who eat 100 grams of soy a day.

Sources

When you include soy in your diet, make sure to eat several different sources of soy. Variety will keep your commitment going, so you don't get bored. Make sure to eat foods that naturally have high amounts of genistein and are not "spiked" by manufacturers who add extra genistein. Also be certain that your soy food is not overprocessed. Micronutrients may be destroyed if food is overprocessed.

The table on page 48 includes a short list of soy foods and the grams of soy protein they contain per standard serving.

Genistein Content of Soy Foods

Tofu, tempeh, miso. If just the sound of soy foods makes you want to say yuck, consider what food scientists are doing. They're engineering foods like burgers, breakfast sausages, and even hot dogs with soy. These are called second-generation soy foods. That's the good news. The bad news is, you may have to eat a lot more of them to get the equivalent amount of genistein. The table on page 49 shows the amount of genistein in the most popular traditional second-generation and soy foods.

Popular Soy Foods

At this time we know from epidemiological studies that the Asian diet lowers rates of heart disease and breast and prostate cancer. So consider the Asian diet as your best means of getting the right amount of soy. In Part III of this book, you

Protein Content of Soy Foods

Food	Serving Size	Gram Weight	Soy Protein (grams)
Miso	1 tablespoon	17	2.0
Soybeans, fresh green	½ cup	90	11.1
Soybeans, mature (dry), cooked	½ cup	86	14.3
Soy flour	1 tablespoon	6	2.6
Soymilk, nonfat*	1 cup	245	6.7
Soy protein powder	1 tablespoon, packed	10	8.1
Tamari soy sauce	1 teaspoon	6	.6
Tempeh	2 ounces	57	10.8
Tofu, baked	2 ounces	57	12
Tofu, firm	2 ounces	57	4.7
Tofu, silken	2 ounces	57	2.7

*Protein content varies; check the label.
Source: USDA

will find easy, prostate-healthy Asian menu plans. Here are other key sources of soy.

Soy Protein Isolate Powder

Protein powder–based soy shakes are the easiest way to eat the large amounts of soy necessary to protect yourself against prostate cancer. You can add the soy protein powder to beverages and blend with fruits to make a delicious, healthy smoothie. On page 141 you'll find a great recipe for a smoothie that contains 20 grams of soy protein. You can also add soy isolate to your cereal or orange juice . . . be creative.

Genistein Content of the Most Popular Foods

Food	Genistein (mg/100 grams)
Soy flakes, defatted	195
Soy flakes, full fat	132
Soy flakes, defatted, toasted	105
Soybean meal, whole	100
Soy flour	94
Soy nuts	94
Soy concentrate, water extracted	91
Soybeans, roasted	87
Soy flour, defatted	75
Soy granules	75
Soybeans, green	73
Soy protein, textured	71
Soybeans, dried	70
Soymilk powder	57
Soy isolate	56
Miso	52
Tofu, dry spiced	42
Tempeh	40
Miso (barley)	34
Tofu, Kikkoman firm	31
Soybean paste	30
Soybean chips	28
Soy isolate, acid	27
Miso (rice)	26
Soybean sprouts	23
Tofu, Àzumaya soft	22
Soy concentrate, alcohol extracted	21
Soy fiber	21
Tofu, Vitasoy silken	21

Food	Genistein (mg/100 grams)
Soybean paste (wheat)	19
Tofu, Nasoya soft	19
Tofu, Tree of Life	19
Tofu, Mori-Ny	18
Tofu	17
Soybean paste (rice)	15
Tofu yogurt	9
Tofu, Weber	9
Soy hot dog	8
Soy bacon	7
Tofu, soft	5
Tofu, firm	5
Soymilk, Banyan	4
Soy cheddar cheese	4
Tofu, fermented	4
Ice Bean	4
Soy mozzarella cheese	4
Soymilk, Plum Flower	3
Soymilk	3
Soymilk formula, Isomil	2
Soy drink, First Alternative	2
Soymilk formula, ProSobee	2
Soy cheese	2
Tofutti	2
Soy concentrate	1
Soy sauce	1
Soy Parmesan	1
Soy-based specialty formula, Enrich	1
Soy-based specialty formula, Jevity	1
Soy-based specialty formula, Glucerna	0

Adapted from *Nutrition and Cancer* 26 (1996): 123–148.

As a powder, the soy protein is more quickly broken down and absorbed. University research teams use concentrate powders in their cancer-prevention trials to ensure that each patient is getting exactly the amount they prescribe.

Brands: Ross Products has a reduced-calcium Health Source Soy Protein Shake Powder, a soy formula used by many prostate cancer patients. Make sure to order reduced-calcium powders, since studies, although still inconclusive, are suggesting that extremely high calcium levels might be implicated in the progression of prostate cancer. Health Source is used in UCSF's prostate cancer study as well as in studies at UCLA for breast cancer. Since this is the product used in careful scientific studies, you have a fair shot of getting the same result if you use this product. Four scoops, or 40 grams a day, of Health Source is the recommended amount. You can order this product at 800-445-3350. In current clinical trials, men are getting a base of 40 grams of soy protein a day with soy isolates, then eating soy-containing foods for the rest. That way they are assured of getting the minimum amount recommended.

Soy protein powder is also available as Vege Fuel from Twin-lab. Genisoy is another popular brand.

Rita Mitchell, R.D., dietitian at the University of California at Berkeley, adds: "Some commercial brands of soy protein powder have additives like sugar or other sweeteners, modified food starches, and other extenders and flavorings. And they are very expensive. We recommend getting it for $3 to $5 a pound in stores where grains and legumes are sold in bulk (as opposed to $15 to $20 a pound for some commercial brands)." If you choose to buy your isolate in bulk, make sure it contains SUPRO. SUPRO, manufactured by Protein

Technologies, is the active ingredient used in *all* good soy isolate powders.

Roasted Soy Nuts

A soy nut snack will fill you up and give you the alerting hit of a good protein. The soy nut is a roasted soybean. The soybean is like a potato. Most of the soybean's mineral value is in the hull. The advantage of whole roasted soy nuts is that they retain the hull. If you're on a very low fat diet, watch the number of soy nuts you eat, since the whole soybean is quite fatty — there are 18.6 grams of fat in ½ cup of dry-roasted, salted soy nuts and 21.8 grams of fat in ½ cup of roasted, salted soy nuts!

Tofu

Tofu is a wonderful soy protein product. It was first used in China in 200 B.C. It is made from soybeans that are washed, soaked, drained, ground, cooked in a soy slurry, and put through a soy milk extractor. A coagulant is added, the product is pressed, the tofu block is cut, and it is packaged, sealed, pasteurized, packed in cases, and put in cold storage.

There are several types of tofu.

- Firm tofu, which is dense and solid, works well with stir-fry dishes or soups. Firm tofu is also the type that is higher in protein, fat, and calcium than the other forms.
- Soft tofu is good for recipes that blend tofu with other ingredients.
- Silken tofu, which is a creamy, custard-like product, works well in blended and pureed dishes.
- Baked tofu is increasingly available in a variety of flavors. Because it has been baked, the moisture has been removed

and it contains more soy protein per serving than fresh tofu. Baked tofu has the consistency of cheese and is great sliced in sandwiches.

Soymilk

This has got to be the easiest way to consume soy protein and takes only a couple of days to get used to. You'll find soymilk refreshing and invigorating. Look for low-fat varieties, since normal soymilk has as much as 4 grams of fat per serving. Soymilk is sometimes called soy drink or soy beverage. Some manufacturers prepare it by soaking soybeans, grinding them, and extracting the liquid. Others mix soy protein isolate with water. Check the Nutrition Facts portion of the food labels. Protein content can vary from 3 to 12 grams per cup, depending on the method of preparation and the brand.

Edamame, or Fresh Green Soybeans

Edamame (ed-uh-MAH-may) is the young, still-green soybean you'll find in Japanese restaurants, where, unfortunately, it's often served heavily salted. Now several Asian food specialty stores and even regular grocery stores carry frozen edamame. You just drop the frozen beans into boiling water for three minutes . . . and they're ready to eat. Be sure not to oversalt them. Some stores even carry fresh, precooked soybeans that you can eat right out of the pod. Don't eat the pod — just pull out the beans. You can also add them to soups or stews or serve them as a vegetable.

Mature (Dry) Soybeans

Dried soybeans are commonly available in bulk in stores where grains and legumes are sold and in some well-stocked grocery stores. If you buy dry soybeans, you'll have to rehydrate them by soaking them in water and then cook them for several hours. They are also becoming more available canned. Mature soybeans are a great source of soy protein.

Soy Tempeh

This is made from cooked soybeans that are fermented, crushed, and formed into cakes. Soy tempeh is great for sandwiches and casseroles. Look for "soy tempeh," as tempeh is made from other grains as well.

Soy Flour

Soybeans may be ground and then processed into a fine flour. Look for soy flour in your health food store.

Second-Generation, or "Engineered," Soy Foods

Food technologists at universities and food companies are scrambling to come up with better-tasting and more convenient soy foods. Soy flour is used in baked goods, and textured soy protein (which begins as soy flour that is compressed to give it a meatier, more granular texture) is used in many veggie burgers. These are called second-generation or engineered soy foods.

Look for soy-based muffins, breads, bakery items, shakes, soups, even pretzels, that are engineered to taste great. Be sure to look at the label, though. Just because these products contain soy protein doesn't mean they are not high in fat.

My favorite soyburger, the Boca Burger, is very tasty, has nearly zero fat, and comes in three different great flavors. The White House orders Boca Burgers; you can now find these burgers at most health food stores and discerning supermarkets. The genistein content of this product, however, has not yet been made public. My favorite Boca product is a breakfast patty that tastes just like real sausage but contains soy protein powder rather than pork!

As you can tell from the table on page 49, second-generation soy foods are not as rich in genistein as traditional soy foods.

In summary, here are some easy sugggestions to increase your soy intake:

- Experiment with many of the soy foods listed in this chapter. A good selection of soy products is becoming more available in many areas of the country. If you don't see what you're looking for, ask the store manager where you shop to stock it for you. They'll be more likely to stock these items if they know there is consumer demand.
- Add cooked soybeans or fresh green soybeans to soups and stews; add soy tempeh to casseroles or spaghetti sauce; add extra tofu to stir fries or soups; add tofu to dishes such as low-fat lasagne. Use silken tofu in deserts such as low-fat chocolate pies.
- Recipe permitting, choose the firmest tofu possible because protein content increases with firmness of the tofu.
- Switch from dairy milk to soymilk.
- Use soy isolate to make shakes.
- Include soy flour in your baked goods. Dr. Barnes suggests that you use no more than 30 percent soy flour replacement, since soy flour does not come with gluten, which is needed to bind the ingredients together.
- Replace meat with soy, e.g., soy burgers.
- Since soy foods can be high in fat, if you actually have

prostate cancer you may want to consider soy protein powders and low-fat soy foods.

For more information on soy, you can contact the Soy Bean Council, a trade group that has a consumer hotline for soy food information and recipes: 800-TALKSOY.

X-Rated Soy Products

These products won't help you fight prostate cancer because they don't have the amount of genistein you need.

Soy Oils

Soy vegetable oil really doesn't shine. It contains 61 percent omega-6 fatty acids. Its hydrogenated form is even worse.

Soy Sauce

Soy sauce is often loaded with sodium and has only a minuscule amount of soy protein. Don't rely on it for anything more than good taste, and even then, be sure you're not ingesting large amounts of sodium. You'll notice the Asian meal plans in this book do contain modest amounts of soy sauce, but at small levels that won't hurt you.

Genistein Supplements

Soy works its magic through its conversion in the gastrointestinal tract, which is why actually eating real soy food is so key. That means real foods work better than supplements. Be sure *not* to take genistein as a supplement by itself until more research is completed and you've discussed it with your doctor. Until then, you're better off sticking with soy foods and high-quality soy powders that fully extract all the key ingredients from soy.

WHAT YOU CAN DO NOW

Include in your diet 40 grams of soy protein a day, but build up to it. Soybeans can cause serious intestinal gas and discomfort, as can any food with high concentrations of soluble fiber. For this reason you will want to start adding soy foods slowly and increase gradually until you've reached the recommended 40 grams. Since you may be eating these foods for years, don't start with an unpleasant experience.

Fats

Aha! What could be better! Aged tenderloin cooked to perfection . . . scrambled eggs and bacon . . . hamburgers barbecued over an open grill. These are among the foods we were brought up believing made us men — red meat, eggs, whole milk, burgers, chops, veal. The great irony is that the very foods we most strongly associate with the All-American-male diet are the ones that put our manhood at greatest risk. Simply stated, fat is the strongest and most consistent nutritional risk for prostate cancer. The evidence goes far beyond simple observation to a detailed biochemical understanding of how fat changes the prostate. You may say, "Oh sure, tell me something new; diets high in fat are bad for you." It's much more interesting than that. Some fats become bioactive. You can think of them as smart bombs, complete with internal guidance that directs them to a pinpoint hit on an exact spot deep inside a prostate cell, which then promotes the growth of cancer. Decades-long exposure to a high-fat diet could explain why prostate cancer increases with increasing age. So if there's one rule to remember about prostate cancer and nutrition, it's this: *The more animal fat you eat, the higher your risk.*[1] While this is a highly controversial point with women and breast cancer, scientists generally agree on it for men with prostate cancer.

Men who consume more than 100 grams of fat a day increase their risk of prostate cancer by as much as 50 percent, reports epidemiologist Dr. Laurence Kolonel of the University of Hawaii. National surveys show that for adult American males, the average daily intake of total fat is about 90 grams in a diet of approximately 2,500 calories — and the majority of that 90 grams is animal fat.

Fat also increases the risk of advanced prostate cancer. Edward Giovannucci, M.D., at Harvard University, found that the more animal fat men ate, the higher their risk of having advanced prostate cancer. The strongest association was with red meat. The data come from a very large study called the Health Professionals Follow-up Study, in which 51,529 U.S. male health professionals aged 40 to 75 completed a validated food-frequency questionnaire in 1986.[2] Follow-up showed that men who ate the most red meat had a risk for advanced prostate cancer 2.64 times greater than men who ate the least red meat. In another study, Richard Hayes, Ph.D., of the National Cancer Institute further confirmed that men who ate more animal fat had a significant increase in risk for cancers that had spread beyond the prostate; in other words, for aggressive cancers.

The most general reason excessive fat can be bad for you is that when the body metabolizes fats, a lot of free radicals are generated. Think of free radicals as political radicals, hacking their way through a fine-china shop with an axe, only the fine china is your DNA. This inflicts what is called "oxidative damage," which can actually create mistakes in your genetic code — and the genetic mistakes or genetic damage make the cells more cancer prone. The day-in, day-out assault on your genes increases the chance of errors that lead to cancer formation or progression. However, cutting-edge research shows that fats have a far more specific action that can affect your risk of getting prostate cancer.

How Can Fats Be Harmful?

The Science

In fascinating new work, scientists are finding fats can strike deep into a prostate cell, directly into the nucleus. The molecular bulls-eye for fats is called a nuclear receptor — in effect, an on-off switch in the heart of the cell.

Nuclear receptors may sound like the punch keypads for secret-strike authorization codes, and you can actually think of them that way. Fats can do their most devastating damage by targeting these nuclear receptors.

The receptor itself is like a specialized lock, and the bioactive fat is the key. Once the fat connects with its receptor, the receptor is turned on and a signal is triggered. Bioactive fats can carry preprogrammed instructions from one part of the body to the other. They deliver that message by locking onto a receptor. What's so intriguing is that there are receptors specialized for different types of fats. That means that the specific kinds of fats you eat may have a direct effect on your risk for cancer. It's almost like taking a drug to achieve a specific effect on the body . . . only instead of a beneficial effect, these fats pose a real threat. Ronald Evans, Ph.D., and Enrike Saez, Ph.D., of the Salk Institute in San Diego have pioneered this promising new area of research. They have honed in on one specific set of receptors that act as fat sensors — receptors called PPARs.

In particular, Dr. Evans and Dr. Saez focused on one of the three receptors in the PPAR family: PPARgamma. PPARgamma can sense the levels of certain fats in the diet; for instance, polyunsaturated fatty acids. Dr. Evans and Dr. Saez showed that PPARgamma *could serve as a molecular link between a high-fat diet and the development of tumors* in the colon. Using an animal model, Dr. Evans and Dr. Saez found that mice fed a normal diet got an average of 1 tumor, whereas mice fed a diet supplemented with a PPARgamma activator developed an average of 3 or more tumors. In other words, activation of PPARgamma led to more tumors.

Dr. Evans and Dr. Saez are now exploring whether PPARgamma plays a role in prostate cancer similar to that in colon cancer. They have fed some mice one diet and the others a diet supplemented with the activator of PPARgamma to examine whether the supplemented diet leads to more prostate cancers or more metastatic cancers. PPARgamma's connection to prostate cancer comes from the fact that PPARgamma is expressed at very high levels in prostate tumors in both humans and mice.

That's the science. Now let's look at fats from a different angle. What kinds of hard observations have been made by epidemiologists to link specific fats to prostate cancer? We'll look at the three basic classes of fats: saturated fats (found in most animal fats), polyunsaturated fats (found in vegetable cooking oils, margarine, fish oils, and many nuts and seeds), and monounsaturated fats (found in olive oil and canola oil). At the end of the chapter we'll look at specific recommendations: which fats to avoid because they may put you at risk and which ones still look safe.

Saturated Fats

The link between fats and prostate cancer is strongest for saturated fats. These are the fats found in fatty meats and whole dairy products, such as milk and cheese. Cardiologists have long warned heart patients to cut down on these fats, as did C. Everett Koop during his tenure as surgeon general. Saturated fat has well earned its reputation as a heart-unhealthy fat. But it was Stanford University's Alice Whittemore, Ph.D., who made the link to prostate cancer and in a very clever way. Her team interviewed 1,500 men with prostate cancer and compared their diets to those of 1,500 men who did not have the disease. The difference? The men with prostate cancer had eaten significantly more saturated fats.

How do saturated fats cause trouble? Scientists suspect it's through their direct effect on male sex hormones. In one study, when researchers reduced fat consumption from 40 percent to 25 percent of total calories, they saw a significant drop in circulating testosterone. Since testosterone may promote prostate cancer growth, a diet low in fat (and high in fiber) could lower testosterone and may therefore reduce cancer growth.

You don't need to wait for the final proof in order to decrease drastically your saturated fat intake — you'll be improving your heart health and your general health as well. There's no downside, and look at the upside. If saturated fat intake *does* increase risk, then, according to Dr. Whittemore's study, Caucasian Americans could eliminate 15 percent of their prostate cancers by eating the same low-fat diet Asians traditionally eat.

For a more extensive list of foods containing saturated fats, see page 63.

Polyunsaturated Fats

Polyunsaturated fats achieved their greatest fame decades ago as a highly promoted substitute for saturated fats. They're found widely in margarines, salad dressings, and vegetable oils such as safflower and corn oils. Many of the polyunsaturated fats are what we call omega-6 fats; some are what we call omega-3 fats. The terms "omega-3" and "omega-6" de-

Saturated Fat Content of Selected Foods

	Serving Size	Weight (grams)	Fat (grams)	Saturated Fat (grams)
Fast Foods				
Cheeseburger, triple patty	1 sandwich	304	51.0	21.7
Hamburger, single patty	1 sandwich	106	9.8	3.6
Fish sandwich with tartar sauce and cheese	1 sandwich	183	28.6	8.1
Chicken fillet sandwich with cheese	1 sandwich	228	38.8	12.4
Burrito with beans	2 pieces	217	13.5	6.9
Burrito with beef and cheese	2 pieces	304	24.8	10.4
Biscuit with egg and bacon	1 biscuit	150	31.1	8.0
Croissant with egg, cheese, and sausage	1 croissant	160	38.2	18.2
French toast sticks	5 pieces	141	29.0	4.7
Hash brown potatoes	½ cup	72	9.2	4.3
Shake, chocolate	1 med. (2 c.)	333	12.3	7.7
Meat, Poultry, and Fish				
Beef, trimmed, lean only, cooked	3 oz.	85	8.6	3.2
Reg. ground beef (27% fat), broiled	3 oz.	85	17.6	6.9
Pork loin, lean only, roasted	3 oz.	85	8.6	3.0
Chicken, light meat, roasted	3 oz.	85	3.8	1.1
Chicken, dark meat, roasted	3 oz.	85	8.7	2.3
Atlantic salmon, cooked	3 oz.	85	6.9	1.1
Rainbow trout, cooked	3 oz.	85	4.9	1.4

	Serving Size	Weight (grams)	Fat (grams)	Saturated Fat (grams)
Meat, Poultry, and Fish, continued				
Halibut, cooked	3 oz.	85	2.5	.4
Tuna, canned in water	3 oz.	85	.7	.2
Shrimp	3 oz. (16 lg.)	85	.9	.2
Whole egg	1 large	50	5.3	1.6
Milk and Dairy Products				
Milk, whole	1 cup	244	8.9	5.6
Milk, 2% fat	1 cup	244	4.7	2.9
Cheese, cheddar	1 oz.	28	9.4	6.0
Cheese, cream	1 oz.	28	9.9	6.2
Cheese, mozzarella	1 oz.	28	4.9	3.1
Cheese, cottage	½ cup	113	4.4	2.8
Yogurt, whole milk	1 cup	245	8.0	5.1
Desserts and Sweets				
Boston cream pie	1 piece	92	7.8	2.2
Cheesecake	1 piece	80	18.0	7.9
Ice cream, full fat	½ cup	74	12.0	7.4
Frozen yogurt	½ cup	72	4.0	2.5
Doughnuts, cake-type	1 doughnut	45	10.3	2.7
Brownie	1 large	56	9.1	2.4
Cookie, chocolate chip	1 large	14	3.2	0.7
Cookie, oatmeal	1 large	18	3.3	0.8

Source: U.S. Department of Agriculture, Agricultural Research Service, 1999. USDA Nutrient Database for Standard Reference, Release 13.

scribe the biochemical makeup of the fat (the 3 and 6 in "omega-3" and "omega-6" refer to the position of the first double bond on the fatty-acid carbon chain). There are three specific polyunsaturated fats that may pose an increased risk for prostate cancer: first, *arachidonic acid,* which is quickly emerging as potentially the most damaging omega-6 fat for prostate cancer risk; second, *linoleic acid,* which has also been implicated, although to a lesser extent; and third, the omega-3 fat *alpha-linolenic acid.* I am including a fourth section on the hazards of polyunsaturated fats called "hydrogenated oils." Fish oils, which are omega-3 fats, have not been linked with increased prostate cancer risk.

Arachidonic Acid

So what is found in a meat-based diet that could lead to cancer but is not found in a vegetarian diet? The answer is arachidonic acid. Arachidonic acid is a polyunsaturated fat found in all meats but especially red meat, dairy fat, and egg yolks. If there is one common denominator in animal fats that is linked to a risk of prostate cancer, it is arachidonic acid.

The case against arachidonic acid: To test whether arachidonic acid is involved in prostate cancer cell growth, the University of Virginia's Charles Myers, M.D., one of the world's top experts on arachidonic acid, took human prostate cancer cells stripped of serum and put them in salt water; ordinarily prostate cancer cells thus treated would die over time. But when Dr. Myers added arachidonic acid, he found that the cells started to grow again. So the arachidonic acid was a strong-enough signal to cause the cells to grow. This observation has been made repeatedly since 1980.

How does a lowly piece of fat acquire the incredible ability to issue sophisticated instructions within the prostate cell? That power is conferred on it by a special conversion to what is called a "bioactive" fat by the name of 5-HETE. That led Dr. Myers to ask what would happen if he blocked that conversion. Sure enough, in an elegant experiment, he blocked the pathway that converts arachidonic acid to 5-HETE. That stopped the prostate cancer cells dead in their tracks — the cancer cells just stopped growing. When Dr. Myers shut down the production of 5-HETE, every prostate cancer cell was dead in two hours! So blocking the production of 5-HETE produced a massive cell death, called apoptosis. Says Dr. Myers: "It is one of the most massive and dramatic forms of apoptosis ever seen in any mammalian cell, benign or malignant." Apoptosis is the process by which cells commit suicide; the cells respond to external signals and then they initiate a genetic program of suicide.[3]

Dr. Myers concluded that arachidonic acid fuels the production of 5-HETE, which in turn fuels both growth and survival of prostate cancer cells. He is now working on developing a drug to target the 5-HETE and cause huge, rapid cancer cell death.

But 5-HETE is not the only product of arachidonic acid that aids in the spread of cancer. Another bioactive fat, called 12-HETE, helps prostate cancer cells invade normal tissues. 12-HETE stimulates the growth of new blood vessels for the tumor. You can see how this could be a fatal combination — increasing the blood vessel growth that allows prostate cancer to spread and cause the growth of more and more cells. How bad is it? Kenneth Honn, Ph.D., of Wayne State University in Detroit and director of the Karmanoss Cancer Institute took human prostate cancer cells that were specially engineered to produce lots of 12-HETE and found that they grew ten times faster because they were able to produce new blood vessels. This study showed the importance of 12-HETE in promoting new blood vessel growth, which helps the cancer move and spread. And advanced cancer *relies* on new blood vessel growth to spread from the prostate. Dr. Honn found that if you inhibit the production of 12-HETE, you can inhibit new blood vessel growth. In animal experiments, he found tumor *regression* when he blocked production of 12-HETE.

Can you reduce levels of arachidonic acid in the blood? Yes! "If someone on a meat diet switches to a vegetarian diet, arachidonic acid levels in the blood will decrease by about 80 percent to 90 percent within a few (2–3) months," says Dr. Myers. He adds that you can't eliminate the last bit of arachidonic acid that remains because it's manufactured by the body itself and is needed for a variety of things, such as blood clotting and control of blood pressure.

Dr. Myers has kindly provided the table below showing

Oils High in Arachidonic Acid Precursors

Oil	% by Oil Weight of Arachidonic Acid Precursor
Safflower	74%
Corn	58%
Cottonseed	52%
Soybean	51%
Peanut	32%

oils high in arachidonic acid precursors. The table is reprinted from Dr. Myers's monthly newsletter *Prostate Forum,* which you can subscribe to by calling 800-305-2432 or 804-974-1303, or visiting the e-mail address www. prostateforum.com.

Linoleic Acid

Linoleic acid is so powerful that when in their experiments scientists want to grow tumors in mice, they put the mice on a corn oil diet, corn oil being a major source of linoleic acid. Linoleic acid is also found in safflower oil, soybean oil, and the cereals, baked foods, and snack foods made with these oils.[4] One study shows that linoleic acid stimulates the growth of prostate cancer in the laboratory. Researchers still want to see further corroboration, though. I've elected to stay away from linoleic acid until more is known.

Alpha-Linolenic Acid

Dr. Edward Giovannucci at Harvard found a positive association between prostate cancer risk and intake of alpha-linolenic acid. Alpha-linolenic acid is found in red meat such as beef, lamb, and pork, and also in mayonnaise, vegetable oils such as soybean or rapeseed oil, and margarine. A Norwegian study verified these findings of a positive association between alpha-linolenic acid and prostate cancer.[5] When Ken Pienta, Ph.D., of the University of Michigan added alpha-linolenic acid to prostate cancer cells in test tubes, he saw a 250 percent increase in the cancer cell growth!

Dr. Myers has kindly provided the table on page 69 showing oils high in alpha-linolenic acid; once again, the table is reprinted from Dr. Myers's monthly newsletter *Prostate Forum.*

Some nuts, such as walnuts, are high in alpha-linolenic

Oils High in Alpha-Linolenic Acid

Oil	% by Oil Weight of Alpha-Linolenic Acid
Linseed	50
Canola	12

acid. The table below gives a more complete list of the alpha-linolenic acid content of certain nuts.

Alpha-linolenic acid may have an upside for other dis-

Alpha-Linolenic Acid in Nuts

Nuts	Grams per Cup
Almonds	0
Cashews	.2
Chestnuts	.1
Hazelnuts	.1
Macadamia nuts	.3
Peanuts	<.1
Pecans	1.2
Pine nuts	.9
Walnuts	10.9

eases. Diets high in this acid have been shown to be heart-healthy and have been linked with a possible reduction in risk of breast and colon cancers. Be aware that some experts contest the alpha-linolenic acid–prostate cancer connection. Until more is known, if you're at high risk you may want to consider reducing your alpha-linolenic acid intake. I stay away from foods high in alpha-linolenic acid in my own diet.

Hydrogenated Oils

The hydrogenation process of a polyunsaturated fat preserves the shelf life of the fat and keeps it solid at room temperature. But transhydrogenated fatty acids can cause DNA damage and increase your cholesterol level and risk of heart disease. You can avoid these fats by carefully reading the ingredient labels when you buy packaged foods. The ingredient list on food products will say "hydrogenated or partially hydro-genated." These are also called transhydrogenated fatty acids. Expect to see soon FDA-required listing of them on labels.

Fish Oils

Eskimos, who eat huge amounts of fish, do have a lower risk of dying of prostate cancer than inland dwellers. Fish con-tains large amounts of fish oil. As tempting as it may seem to link fish oil with cancer prevention, there is no other evidence linking fish oils with decreased prostate cancer growth or risk. Dr. Dean Ornish recommends 2 to 3 grams a day of fish oil for the cardioprotective effects but does not yet include them in his landmark study of lifestyle intervention in prostate cancer patients. Dr. Charles Myers has preliminary data suggesting that flaxseed oil but not fish oil may promote the growth of prostate cancer. The good news is that epi-demiological studies show no added risk from eating actual fish as opposed to the oils. And fish oils are the heart-healthiest fats. If you are trying to cut your fat intake, limit your con-sumption of high-fat fish such as mackerel, tuna canned in oil, salmon, and trout. Instead, choose lower-fat white fish such as cod, halibut, and tuna canned in water, or clams, crab, scallops, shrimp, or lobster.

Avoiding fish and just taking 2 to 3 grams a day of fish oil capsules gives you the benefits of the omega-3 fatty acids without the fat and arachidonic acid found in fish.

Monounsaturated Fats

Monounsaturated fat is oleic acid, which is an omega-9 fat. The best food source of monounsaturated fat is olive oil. Let's look at it.

Olive Oil

If you're going to eat a fat and want to be reasonably certain there's not even a tenuous link to prostate cancer, olive oil is it. But don't go overboard — remember, you're trying to keep your total fat intake low and a tablespoon has 14 grams of fat! There's no evidence establishing protective benefits of olive oil for prostate cancer risk, but there's also no evidence that it is of any harm to the prostate, something that's hard to say about most fats. Still, olive oil does contain some saturated fat and is not considered completely prostate healthy by Dr. Dean Ornish.

Fats' Other Danger: Calories

Fat is the most dense form of calories and provides the greatest number of calories in the body. One gram of fat provides 9 calories! François Meyer, M.D., Ph.D., professor at Laval University, found that the more calories you eat, the higher the chance that you will have an indolent cancer, whereas the more saturated fat you eat, the greater your risk of later-stage disease. "There *is* a relation between total energy intake and incidental prostate cancer or occult cancers. Greater total energy intake was associated with greater occurrence of occult cancers." This suggested that two separate dietary influences may be affecting different parts of the development of prostate cancer: total energy intake may play a role in early development, while fat intake plays a role in the tumor's transition to clinically important cancer.

A low-calorie diet slows the progress of prostate cancer in animals, new research shows. The slowing of tumor progression occurred whether the calories were reduced by cutting fat, carbohydrates, or the overall diet. The results further suggested the way that the lower-calorie diet slowed tumor growth in rats and mice — it retarded the development of new blood vessels in the tumor. The research was conducted at the Ohio State University Comprehensive Cancer Center.

On page 73 is a table showing the fat content of some popular foods.

WHAT YOU CAN DO NOW
If You're at High Risk

Consider decreasing your total fat intake to just 10 percent of calories. That's the mark set in current clinical trials. To get your fat intake to a bare minimum, avoid all oils, avocado, nuts, olives, and almonds. The Asian menu plans on page 142 have been designed to keep your fat intake at about 10 percent of calories. Since there are huge variations in the amount of activity that men undertake, depending on where they stand, from triathletes to pencil jockeys, there is no recommended number of calories per day. Try to carve out some time with a nutritionist to see how many calories you really need for your lifestyle.

Fat Content of Selected Popular Foods

	Serving Size	Weight (grams)	Fat (grams)
Grains			
Cereal, puffed wheat	1 cup	12	.2
Cereal, crispy rice	1 cup	28	.1
Cereal, shredded wheat	1 oblong biscuit	25	.4
Cereal, granola, homemade	¼ cup	30	7.5
Cereal, oatmeal, cooked	½ cup	117	1.2
Bulgur, cooked	½ cup	91	.2
Bread, whole wheat	1 slice	28	1.2
Bread, white	1 slice	25	.9
Crackers, graham	2 squares	14	1.4
Crackers, saltines	5 squares	15	1.7
Crackers, melba toast	5 melba rounds	15	.5
Crackers, whole wheat	3 crackers	12	2.1
Soy Products			
Mature (dry) soybeans, cooked	½ cup	86	7.7
Baked tofu	2 ounces	57	1.3
Fresh green soybeans	½ cup	90	5.8
Soy tempeh	2 ounces	57	4.4
Firm tofu	2 ounces	57	2.5
Soy protein powder	1 tbsp., packed	10	.3
Nonfat soymilk	1 cup	245	0
Silken tofu	2 ounces	57	1.5

	Serving Size	Weight (grams)	Fat (grams)
Snack Foods			
Potato chips, plain	1 ounce	28	9.8
Pretzels, plain	5 twists	30	1.1
Popcorn, air-popped	1 cup	8	.3
Popcorn, oil-popped	1 cup	11	3.1
Trail mix	¼ cup	37	11.6
Granola bar, soft, uncoated	1 bar	28	4.9
Desserts and Sweets			
Angel food cake	1 piece	50	.2
Boston cream pie	1 piece	92	7.8
Cheesecake	1 piece	80	18.0
Ice cream, full fat	½ cup	74	12.0
Ice cream, reduced fat	½ cup	66	2.8
Sherbet	½ cup	74	1.5
Fruit ices	½ cup	99	0
Frozen yogurt	½ cup	72	4.0
Doughnuts, cake-type	1 doughnut	45	10.3
Brownie	1 large	56	9.1
Cookie, chocolate chip	1 large	14	3.2
Cookie, fig bar	1 bar	16	1.2
Cookie, oatmeal	1 large	18	3.3
Cookie, vanilla wafer	1 wafer	6	1.2
Meat, Poultry, and Fish			
Beef, trimmed, lean only, cooked	3 oz.	85	8.6

	Serving Size	Weight (grams)	Fat (grams)
Meat, Poultry, and Fish, continued			
Beef, trimmed, lean and fat, cooked	3 oz.	85	20.0
Extra lean ground beef (17% fat), broiled	3 oz.	85	13.9
Regular ground beef (27% fat), broiled	3 oz.	85	17.6
Pork loin, lean only, roasted	3 oz.	85	8.6
Bologna	1 med. slice	28	8.0
Chicken, light meat, meat only, roasted	3 oz.	85	3.8
Chicken, light meat, meat and skin, roasted	3 oz.	85	9.2
Chicken, dark meat, meat only, roasted	3 oz.	85	8.7
Chicken, dark meat, meat and skin, roasted	3 oz.	85	13.4
Atlantic salmon, cooked	3 oz.	85	6.9
Rainbow trout, cooked	3 oz.	85	4.9
Halibut, cooked	3 oz.	85	2.5
Tuna, canned in water	3 oz.	85	.7
Swordfish	3 oz.	85	4.3
Shrimp	3 oz. (16 large)	85	.9
Crab	3 oz.	85	.8
Whole egg	1 large	50	5.3
Egg white	1 large	33	0
Egg yolk	1 large	17	5.1

	Serving Size	Weight (grams)	Fat (grams)
Milk and Dairy Products			
Milk, whole	1 cup	244	8.9
Milk, 2% fat	1 cup	244	4.7
Milk, skim	1 cup	245	.6
Cheese, cheddar	1 oz.	28	9.4
Cheese, cheddar, low fat	1 oz.	28	2.0
Cheese, cream	1 oz.	28	9.9
Cheese, mozzarella	1 oz.	28	4.9
Cheese, cottage	½ cup	113	4.4
Yogurt, whole milk	1 cup	245	8.0
Yogurt, skim milk	1 cup	245	.4
Fast Foods			
Cheeseburger, triple patty	1 sandwich	304	51.0
Hamburger, single patty	1 sandwich	106	9.8
Fish sandwich with tartar sauce and cheese	1 sandwich	183	28.6
Chicken fillet sandwich with cheese	1 sandwich	228	38.8
Burrito with beans	2 pieces	217	13.5
Burrito with beef and cheese	2 pieces	304	24.8
Biscuit with egg and bacon	1 biscuit	150	31.1
Croissant with egg, cheese, and sausage	1 croissant	160	38.2
French toast sticks	5 pieces	141	29.0
Hash brown potatoes	½ cup	72	9.2
Shake, chocolate	1 med. (2 cups)	333	12.3

	Serving Size	Weight (grams)	Fat (grams)
Fats and Oils			
Butter	1 pat	5	4.1
Margarine	1 teaspoon	5	3.8
Mayonnaise	1 tablespoon	14	11.0
Italian salad dressing	1 tablespoon	15	7.1
Italian salad dressing, diet	1 tablespoon	15	1.5
Oils	1 tablespoon	14	14

Amount of fat in a tablespoon: A tablespoon of any kind of oil has approximately 120 calories. A teaspoon is about ⅓ of a tablespoon, so it's about 40 calories.

Here's how the calculation is done. All oils are 100% fat, and 1 gram of fat always provides the same number of calories: 9 calories per gram. A tablespoon of oil weighs approximately 13.5–14 grams, and 13.5 grams of fat multiplied by 9 calories provides approximately 120 calories.

Source: U.S. Department of Agriculture, Agricultural Research Service, 1999. USDA Nutrient Database for Standard Reference, Release 13.

If You're at Low to Moderate Risk

If you don't have prostate cancer and are not at high risk but want to manage what risk you do have, you'll want to consider reducing your intake of fat to a minimum. How much total fat? Dr. Myers says: "Twenty percent, and if you can go the extra distance to ten percent, that's better. It takes a lean horse for a long race."

- Use foods from plant sources (whole grains, vegetables, fruits, and legumes) as the foundation for most meals.
- Model your diet on a vegetarian or Asian or low-fat, fish-based diet.
- Use cooking methods that don't require the use of added fat.

For this, you'll find a good nonstick skillet indispensable.
- Avoid the saturated fats in animal meat, dairy, and eggs.
- Limit obvious sources of fat, such as commercial salad dressings, mayonnaise, cream sauces, whipping cream, and other dessert toppings.
- Reduce or eliminate your intake of corn oil, vegetable oil, and margarine.
- Avoid hydrogenated oils.
- Be aware of the foods with "invisible fat" that increase your fat intake. These include snack foods such as chips and many crackers, fried foods, nuts and seeds, and nondairy creamers.
- Choose fruit desserts and ices instead of high-fat cakes, pies, and pastries.
- When fat is needed, use olive oil.

The Mediterranean menu plans on page 157 have been designed to keep your fat intake at about 15 to 20 percent of calories.

Special note on low-fat diets: Some men don't do well on a low-fat diet, largely because it is the wrong low-fat diet. Here's what happens. A diet in which refined flours and sugars replace fats can have an untoward effect on blood-fat levels. Triglycerides in particular can rise if poor-quality carbohydrates are substituted for fat. If you find yourself in the unenviable situation in which your blood-fat levels are adversely affected by a low-fat diet, read the chapter on insulin to be sure you've limited the carbohydrates that drive up blood-sugar levels. If that doesn't work and your doctor feels you need to eat more fat, then consider olive oil and fish as your heart-healthiest choices. Also, if you just plain won't eat a low-fat diet, consider a Mediterranean-style diet that uses these "good" fats (although this may not go far enough if you already have prostate cancer or are at high risk for it).

Antioxidants

The word antioxidant is so overused I wonder it's not used in toothpaste ads. Or that there isn't a spoof advertisement like the one you may have seen for a popular health bar. Picture a crusty old New Englander grumbling, "What in hell's an antioxidant?" The ubiquitous nature of the word makes many of us tend to ignore it. But behind all the jargon is a concept that is critical to cancer prevention. Here's why.

Just as an automobile engine generates exhaust even at idle, so, too, cells in the human body generate exhaust. While automobile exhaust may contain carbon monoxide and other toxins, your cells also produce highly toxic substances, the worst of which is called an oxygen free radical. These molecules are "damagers," wreaking havoc in the cell by creating what is called "oxidative damage." Cells in our body are generating oxidative damage all the time. Oxygen free radical molecules set up a harmful mini chain reaction. These molecules first attack the cell's wall. And that's where the real trouble lurks. Fatty acids make up the cell wall, and once these fats are "oxidized," they help launch strikes deep within the cell to attack the cell's genetic machinery, namely DNA. Damaged DNA is prone to mutate. This substantially increases the chances of the cell becoming cancerous. There are several studies showing a correlation between oxidative damage and cancer growth. That makes blocking oxidative damage a cornerstone of cancer prevention. If you could block the initial event, you might actually prevent the cancer from beginning.

The oxygen free radical is a *pro*oxidant. The good news

is, it can be counteracted with an *anti*oxidant. "My hypothesis is that the balance in the cell environment of prooxidants and antioxidants is very important for cancer cell growth," says Neil Fleshner, M.D., urologic oncologist and expert on oxidation at the University of Toronto. "Oxidative damage causes oncogenes to be produced or expressed in the cell. If this hypothesis is true, then things that increase oxidative stress should be bad for prostate cancer and antioxidants should protect against prostate cancer."

Fat provides the raw material for oxidative damage. When fats become unstable, they generate free radicals. That's why a high-fat diet may increase cell damage. But diet is not alone as a risk factor for oxidative damage.

There are other factors related to oxidative stress and implicated in prostate cancer. Oxidative damage can also be thought of like the rusting of an old car, and several lifestyle factors can contribute to that rusting. The four clear factors that affect oxidative stress are: smoking, sedentary lifestyle, aging, and male sex hormones, all of which increase cell oxidation through a host of mechanisms.[1]

The prostate is especially prone to this oxidative stress. Why? Prostate cells have an Achilles' heel. It's an enzyme called cyclooxygenase. The human prostate contains large amounts of cyclooxygenase, which can generate a ton of free radicals.

How do you lower your oxidative load? There are two effective ways of lowering oxidative load. The first is by decreasing fats in the diet, not smoking, and increasing activity. The second is by ingesting enormously powerful antioxidants, and that is the heart of this chapter. Antioxidants block or "mop up" the oxygen free radicals. Let's take a look at the key antioxidants that can help your body mop up oxygen free radicals.

Specific Antioxidants

One pet peeve I have about reading cancer prevention books is that they seem to have an exhaustive list of vitamins, minerals, antioxidants, and other substances none of which is more important than the other, which gives you little motivation to embrace them. What's so satisfying about nutrition in prostate cancer is that there is a handful of foods and supplements with highly specific and advantageous benefits. I have rated them from five stars (★★★★★) down to one star (★) for their effectiveness and degree of scientific validation.

★★★★ *Vitamin E*

Vitamin E is the premier fat-soluble vitamin for prostate cancer prevention. The most intriguing evidence comes from a Finnish study called the ATBC Trial. Researchers weren't even looking for prostate cancer risk; they were trying to determine if vitamin E or beta-carotene worked to protect participants from lung cancer. (They didn't!) But there was a stunning and totally unexpected finding. Participants who took vitamin E had a 30 percent reduced risk of diagnosis of prostate cancer and a 40 percent reduced death rate from prostate cancer. Researchers are now feverishly working to prove, in a more direct fashion, the protective benefit of vitamin E against prostate cancer. While we're waiting for the conclusive findings, increasing your intake of vitamin E–rich foods makes a lot of sense. Whole grains and green leafy vegetables are great sources of vitamin E. If you want to take vitamin E as a supplement, don't overdo it. A lot of vitamin E could cause bleeding and might pose a danger of stroke. In the Finnish trial, benefit was seen with just 50 IU per day; and you could easily get that amount from a multivitamin.

★★★★★ *Selenium*

Selenium, a mineral found in the soil, has been shown — like vitamin E, quite by accident — to prevent prostate cancer growth. Dr. Larry Clark, at the University of Arizona, had set up a trial for selenium and skin cancer. This trial included 1,300 subjects at risk for skin cancer (they were living in Arizona and already had one skin cancer). Half the group got selenium (200 micrograms once a day), and the other half got a placebo. Dr. Clark ran the study for eight years. At the end of the study, he saw no effect for selenium on skin cancer. But he discovered that the group that took selenium had a 50 percent reduction in prostate cancer diagnosis! (The study also showed a 50 percent reduction in lung cancer and colon cancer.) There may be hidden biases in this study, since the study was focusing on skin cancer, but Dr. Clark's findings nevertheless spurred a flurry of studies that have been confirming the benefit of selenium in preventing prostate cancer.

At Harvard, Walter Willett, M.D., measured selenium blood samples and found that having low amounts of selenium in the bloodstream was linked to higher rates of prostate cancer. Edward Giovannucci, M.D., also at Harvard, examined the selenium content of toenail clippings — the selenium in toenails correlates with the amount of selenium in the bloodstream. And Dr. Giovannucci found that the group with the lowest amount of selenium had double the risk of prostate cancer. In his selenium study, Dr. James Brooks, urologic oncologist at Stanford University, replicated Dr. Giovannucci's findings and again established that men with the lowest levels of selenium in their bloodstream had twice the risk of prostate cancer as men with the highest selenium levels.

Dr. Clark is now preparing to repeat the selenium trial, this time with prostate cancer patients. And the National Cancer Institute is organizing a 32,000-man study that will investigate prostate cancer prevention with vitamin E and selenium.

Exactly how selenium works is still unclear, but research is pointing to effective antioxidant activity. Scientists have found that men with more selenium had higher concentrations of an enzyme called the phase-2 enzyme glutathione peroxidase. The current hypothesis is that glutathione peroxidase eliminates oxygen free radicals; in other words, it's an antioxidant.

Selenium is taken up by foods from the soil as they grow. Selenium is found in grains and in the animals eating these grains. Still, selenium is difficult to get from foods, but can be found in grains and garlic grown in soil rich in selenium. Garlic does not normally contain a lot of selenium, but grown in a selenium-rich soil it absorbs a good deal. You can find selenized yeast in health food stores. Selenium can also be taken as a supplement.

★★★ Green Tea

Green tea has one of the highest antioxidant values known. The antioxidants in green tea are called polyphenols. One polyphenol, epigallocatechin gallate (EGCG), has been shown in cell cultures to be a more powerful antioxidant than vitamin E or vitamin C. One study showed EGCG to prevent cancer growth and lower cholesterol.[2] Another study found that drinking 3 to 10 cups of green tea a day is related to fewer numbers of certain cancers.[3]

Green tea is now being tested in clinical trials for prostate cancer prevention. The usual recommended dose is 4 cups a day in these trials. Although there is little data specific to prostate cancer, I still try to drink the equivalent of 4 cups of green tea a day. Some studies suggest that black tea works as well as green tea.

★★★★★ Vegetables and Fruits

In addition to incorporating the antioxidants listed above in your diet, following a diet high in vegetables and fruits is the most powerful proactive step you can take to lower oxidant load. These foods also displace starches to cut glucose load. The National Cancer Institute recommends to all adults 5 to 9 helpings of vegetables *and* fruits per day.

Intake of vegetables and fruits should be distributed throughout the day. Here's why. Oxidant load is reduced as soon as food is eaten and digested because the nutrients are absorbed into the blood.

Antioxidant potential: The tables on pages 86 and 87 show the ability of fruits and vegetables to act as antioxidants. The actual values are expressed as antioxidant capacity.

Garlic tops the list of foods able to absorb oxygen radicals. The more foods you eat from the top of the list, the better. I'm always asked about garlic by men concerned about prostate cancer. Is there anything special about it? Garlic is very promising and is being tested not only for slowing down the growth of prostate cancer, but also for preventing its onset. Include garlic in your vegetable dishes or tomato sauces; turn to the recipes sections of this book (pages 146, 154, and 161) to find how to incorporate garlic in healthy, delicious recipes. Most experts believe you should get your garlic from foods, not pills. The good news is that palate-friendly vegetables such as garlic, kale, onions, corn, and sweet potatoes, and delicious fruits, such as strawberries,

Antioxidant Capacity of Selected Fruits

Fruit	Antioxidant Capacity
Strawberry	15.36
Plum	9.49
Orange	7.50
Grape, red	7.39
Kiwifruit	6.02
Grapefruit, pink	4.83
Grape, white	4.46
Banana	2.21
Apple	2.18
Tomato	1.89
Pear	1.34
Melon	0.97

Adapted with permission from *Journal of Agricultural and Food Chemistry* 44 (1996): 701–705. Copyright © 1996 American Chemical Society.

plums, oranges, and red grapes, are so high on the list of antioxidants.

Phytosterols: Vegetables, including vegetable salads and beans, also contain phytosterols. Plants store phytosterols in an oil form in their membranes. There are several phytosterols, but the two main ones are beta-sitosterol and campesterol.

Atif Awad, Ph.D., of the University of Buffalo found that beta-sitosterol inhibited the growth of prostate cancer cells.

If you eat salads, increase your vegetable intake, and cut down on animal fat in your diet, you'll increase the amount of phytosterols in your body. Vegetarians and Asians ingest around 400 milligrams of phytosterols a day from their diet; Americans average 80 milligrams of phytosterols a day in

Antioxidant Capacity of Selected Vegetables

Vegetable	Antioxidant Capacity
Garlic	19.4
Kale	17.7
Spinach	12.6
Brussels sprouts	9.8
Alfalfa sprouts	9.3
Broccoli florets	8.9
Beets	8.4
Red bell pepper	7.1
Onion	4.5
Corn	4.0
Eggplant	3.9
Cauliflower	3.8
Potato	3.1
Sweet potato	3.0
Cabbage	3.0
Leaf lettuce	2.6
Carrot	2.1
String beans	2.0
Yellow squash	1.5
Iceberg lettuce	1.2
Celery	0.6
Cucumber	0.5

Adapted with permission from *Journal of Agricultural and Food Chemistry* 44 (1996): 3426–3431. Copyright © 1996 American Chemical Society.

their diet. And Americans have high levels of cholesterol, while Asians have low levels of cholesterol.

All plants have phytosterols; you can use the table on page 89 to help you choose phytosterol-rich foods.

Some experts argue that there is no clear evidence that fruits offer any benefit for decreasing prostate cancer risk. I still eat lots of fruits but choose those that have the highest amounts of antioxidants.

If you think you already have enough fruits and vegetables in your diet, think again! A national survey conducted by the National Cancer Institute (NCI) in 1991 showed that the average intake of fruits and vegetables in the U.S. was 3.5 servings a day. Only 36 percent of the U.S. population were aware that they should be eating at least 5 helpings of fruits and vegetables a day, and only 23 percent reported consuming the minimum recommendations. Although the analysis from a 1997 follow-up study is not complete, Dr. Linda Nebeling at NCI says that "from the preliminary analysis it does not look like the consumption figures have improved very significantly. The problem is that people are eating processed foods and meats and simplified sources of carbohydrates. They are getting more than the adequate calories, but not the right balance of nutrients." The next two antioxidants, sulforaphane and lycopene, are found in vegetables.

★★★★★ *Sulforaphane*

While we commonly think of foods and vitamins as containing antioxidants, the body also makes its own antioxidants. We can help our bodies make many more of their own antioxidants with a compound called sulforaphane, which has

Phytosterol Content of Foods

The table below shows the total phytosterol, beta-sitosterol, and campesterol content of foods. The total phytosterol figure is a reflection of *all* the sterols in the food, not just the beta-sitosterol and campesterol numbers combined. You should select foods high in beta-sitosterol and total sterol.

Food	Total Sterol	Beta-sitosterol	Campesterol
	(mg/100 grams edible portions)		
Vegetables			
Bamboo shoots	19	15	3
Barley seedlings, dry	234	98	33
Beans:			
kidney, with pods, immature	14	7	1
mung, sprouts	15	5	1
Beets:			
greens	21	13	tr*
root	25		
Brussels sprouts	24	17	6
Cabbage	11	7	2
Carrots	12	7	1
Cauliflower	18	12	3
Celery	6	2	tr
Chives	9	7	1
Cucumber	14	14	
Eggplant	7	3	tr
Garlic, Chinese	1	1	tr
Ginger root	15	10	1
Gourds:			
bottle	9	5	_**

Food	Total Sterol	Beta-sitosterol	Campesterol
	(mg/100 grams edible portions)		

Vegetables, continued

Food	Total Sterol	Beta-sitosterol	Campesterol
wax	7	5	–
white, dry	119	89	2
Lettuce:			
garden	38	21	2
head	10	5	1
Jerusalem artichokes (interior, dry)	23		
Mustard greens:			
brown	6	5	1
Chinese	2	2	tr
potherb	4	3	1
Okra	24	15	3
Onion	15	12	1
Parsley	5	2	tr
Pepper:			
red	13	7	3
sweet	9	6	2
Potato:			
sweet	12	8	3
white	5	3	tr
Pumpkin	12	12	–
Radish:			
greens	34	22	6
root	11	6	5
Shallots	5	4	tr
Soybeans, immature	50	30	9

Food	Total Sterol	Beta-sitosterol	Campesterol
		(mg/100 grams edible portions)	

Vegetables, continued

Food	Total Sterol	Beta-sitosterol	Campesterol
Spinach	9	–	tr
Taro	19	11	3
Tomato	7	3	1
Turnip:			
greens	12	9	2
root	7	5	1
Vetch, dry	52		
Yam	10	7	2

Legumes

Food	Total Sterol	Beta-sitosterol	Campesterol
Beans:			
azuki	76	37	1
broad	124	95	8
kidney	127	91	3
mung	23	13	2
sasage	99	43	6
Peas:			
chickpea	35		
common	135	106	10
Soybeans	161	90	23

Fruits

Food	Total Sterol	Beta-sitosterol	Campesterol
Apple	12	11	1
Apricot	18	16	1
Banana	16	11	2
Cherry	12	12	tr

Food	Total Sterol	Beta-sitosterol	Campesterol
	(mg/100 grams edible portions)		

Fruits, continued

Food	Total Sterol	Beta-sitosterol	Campesterol
Fig	31	27	1
Grape	4	3	tr
Grapefruit	17	13	2
Lemon:			
whole	12	8	2
peelings	35	22	4
Loquat	2	2	tr
Muskmelon	10	8	–
Orange:			
navel	24	17	4
peelings, navel	34	26	4
Peach	10	6	1
Pear	8	7	–
Persimmon	4	3	–
Pineapple	6	4	1
Plum	7	6	tr
Pomegranate	17	16	tr
Strawberries	12	10	tr
Watermelon	2	1	tr

Cereals

Food	Total Sterol	Beta-sitosterol	Campesterol
Buckwheat	198	164	20
Corn	178	120	32
Oats, dry	58		
Rice bran	1,325	735	257
Sorghum	178	97	35

	Total Sterol	Beta-sitosterol	Campesterol
Food		(mg/100 grams edible portions)	
Cereals, continued			
Wheat:			
bran (hard wheat)	154		
bran (soft wheat)	89		
flour	60		

*tr = trace amounts (<0.5 mg sterol)
**Dashes (–) = not detected
Adapted with permission from *Journal of the American Dietetic Association* 73 (July 1978): 44–45. Copyright © The American Dietetic Association.

been shown to have antitumor activity. Cruciferous vegetables — such as broccoli, Brussels sprouts, cabbage, cauliflower, or kale — all contain sulforaphane.

The body's own antioxidants: The most important of the body's own antioxidants for prostate cancer are called phase-2 enzymes. Phase-2 enzymes all do the same thing: they detoxify carcinogens and turn them into water-soluble substances that can be excreted by the cell. Scientists have long known that all phase-2 enzymes are important and that the loss of even one can raise your risk of cancer.

The GSTP1 enzyme: GSTP1 is a phase-2 enzyme that is universally absent in prostate cancer cells but present in normal prostate tissue. GSTP1 (glutathione S-transferase-π) is very good at detoxifying both oxidants and actual carcinogens. However, one study shows that when GSTP1 is working poorly, men are at an increased risk for prostate cancer. And in cancer cells, GSTP1 is completely absent. "Prostate cancers, breast cancers, and liver cancers all seem to inactivate GSTP1," says William Nelson, M.D., Ph.D., oncologist and antioxidation expert at Johns Hopkins University.

"GSTP1 is lost in prostate cancer probably because it's turned off," suggests Dr. Brooks.

How to turn on your body's own antioxidants: The key question now is how to compensate for the loss of GSTP1. Dr. Brooks says: "There is a lot of evidence going back to the 1950s that shows that you can turn on the phase-2 enzymes." And compounds found in certain foods seem to be protective — "all indications are that sulforaphane, a compound found in broccoli and other cruciferous vegetables, is the most potent compound for turning on the phase-2 enzymes," says Dr. Brooks.

Sulforaphane was discovered by Paul Talalay, M.D., at Johns Hopkins when he and his colleagues were looking for a substance in cruciferous vegetables that would raise phase-2 enzymes. "We wanted to boost the phase-2 enzymes." Phase-2 enzymes detoxify carcinogenic chemicals such as nitrosamine. Says Dr. Talalay, "It was our hypothesis, subsequently confirmed, that if you were able to raise phase-2 enzymes, you would establish a resistance to cancer. The important principle was that if something raised the detoxification enzymes, that would result in protection against carcinogens."

Dr. Talalay studied vegetables and found that some, such as broccoli and other cruciferous vegetables, were rich in the detoxification activity. In addition to sulforaphane, he also found glucoraphanin, which is the precursor of the sulforaphane found in cruciferous vegetables.

Glucoraphanin: When Dr. Talalay and his colleagues administered sulforaphanes to mammary tumors in rats, they saw a huge protective strategy. There was a marked reduction (at least 50%) in the incidence of tumors, the multiplicity (i.e., number) of tumors, the size, and the development of tumors. Dr. Talalay also found that 3-day-old sprouts of arugula, bok choy, broccoli, cabbage, cauliflower, Chinese cabbage, collards, cress, daikon, kale, kohlrabi, mustard, turnip, and watercress had 10 to 100 times more glucoraphanin than corresponding mature plants. Broccoli sprouts especially were highly effective in reducing the incidence of cancer, and the multiplicity and rate of development of the tumors.[4]

Cruciferous vegetables have in common a crosslike leaf. Examples include:

bok choy	collard	mustard seed
broccoli	cress	rutabaga
Brussels sprouts	horseradish	turnip
cabbage	kale	
cauliflower	kohlrabi	

Since Dr. Talalay's studies have so far concentrated on the pharmacology of broccoli sprouts, he is now conducting human studies to establish whether consumption of broccoli sprouts in human volunteers will raise levels of phase-2 enzymes and protect against oxidative stress. These human studies are at an early stage, but Dr. Talalay says there's no need to wait — incorporating broccoli sprouts in your diet will not hurt and may help protect you.

Sprouts: When Dr. Talalay looked at mature broccoli, he couldn't tell which samples had more glucoraphanin than others. He discovered that young cruciferous plants, such as broccoli sprouts, could contain exceedingly high concentrations of glucoraphanin — 20 to 50 times more than supermarket broccoli samples, which themselves varied enormously! This is important because most individuals cannot consume the large quantities of cruciferous vegetables required to lower cancer risk, so sprouts offer a great alternative.

Broccoli sprouts contain much higher levels of glucoraphanin, so you can eat less of them than broccoli to get the same amount of glucoraphanin. The sprouts do not taste like mature broccoli. They are rather tangy, sharp — a taste which is very pleasant. They can be incorporated into salads or sandwiches or just eaten by themselves. Because of possible E-coli contamination, raw sprouts should not be eaten by children, the elderly, and individuals with compromised immune systems. As this book goes to press, an FDA advisory recommends that all people who want to reduce the risk of food-borne illnesses from sprouts should *not* eat raw sprouts. This does not take away from the benefits of uncontaminated sprouts. Before you include raw sprouts in your diet, consult with your doctor.

Broccoli sprouts can be made to a standard. Dr. Talalay and his colleague, plant physiologist Dr. Jed W. Fahey, have a patent on broccoli sprouts that contain high levels of sulforaphane or glucoraphanin. The patent belongs to Johns Hopkins. These Johns Hopkins broccoli sprouts are called BroccoSprouts and are sold under that name in various parts of the country. BroccoSprouts have been analyzed for sulforaphane contents in commercial labs. The company making them is called Brassica Sprout Group and is located in Minneapolis. Since other broccoli sprouts may or may not contain adequate amounts of the sulforaphane precursor, you may want to call the Brassica

Sprout Group to find out where in your area you can buy Broc-coSprouts (phone number: 410-837-9244).

Dr. Talalay and his colleagues are now working on establishing a recommended dose of broccoli sprouts per day for humans. They don't have an answer yet, but they do know that when consuming broccoli sprouts, we need to eat only 1/20 of the amount of mature broccoli. So eating 2 servings of broccoli sprouts per day is comparable to eating 40 servings of mature broccoli!

Warning:
• Fresh versus frozen broccoli. Fresh broccoli is 6 to 7 times as effective as frozen broccoli. During the freezing process, broccoli passes through a steam that does two things: it reduces bacterial contamination, and kills the enzymes that give broccoli an off-flavor. This freezing process, Dr. Talalay and other experts believe, leaches out some of the beneficial presulforaphane compounds.

• Avoid wilted vegetables since the heat that caused the wilting will also have deactivated some of the beneficial compounds.

• Studies have shown that you have to eat the actual fresh vegetables — supplements of dried vegetables are not as efficient.

Other benefits: A few epidemiological studies suggest that about a half pound of mature broccoli per day would reduce colon cancer risk by 50 percent, but no such studies exist for prostate cancer.

★★★★★ Lycopene

Lycopene is a carotenoid. Carotenoids are the pigments that give vegetables and fruits their colors such as green, yellow, and red. Lycopene gives tomatoes their red color. Carotenoids have strong antioxidant and anticancer qualities. Studies show that lycopene is most likely the carotenoid responsible for the protection against heart disease and cancer which had long been credited to another carotenoid, beta-carotene. Since lycopene is such a powerful antioxidant and is being so heavily tested for its anti–prostate cancer properties, you'll find the entire following chapter devoted to it.

★★★★★ *Genistein*

A substance produced by the soybean, genistein has many remarkable cancer-fighting properties. Genistein is also a very powerful antioxidant. You'll find lots more on genistein in the chapter on soy (page 40).

WHAT YOU CAN DO NOW
Fruits and Vegetables

- If you really want to drop your oxidative load, nine servings of vegetables and fruits a day is the way to go. That's the maximum recommended by the National Cancer Institute. While that sounds like a lot, vegetables are an excellent source of minerals, vitamins, and other key nutrients. You're also getting the greatest number of nutrients for the fewest number of calories. These foods are high in the fibers that fight hunger and will naturally displace fats and refined carbohydrates in your diet. With nine a day, blood levels of carotenoids can double in healthy people. It takes about six days to hit peak blood levels after you change your diet.
- Choose fruits and vegetables from the top of the antioxidation tables on pages 86 and 87 to get the greatest amount of antioxidants.

- Drink one (6-ounce) serving of canned tomato juice and eat at least one other serving of tomato food per day.
- To get the full effect of genistein, aim for 40 grams of soy protein in your diet.
- Eat 2 servings of cruciferous vegetables a day, such as baby broccoli.
- Increase your intake of phytosterol to 400 milligrams a day by choosing foods high in phytosterols from the chart on page 89.
- Drink 4 cups of green tea a day.
- Increase your intake of vitamin E through foods.

Supplements

You can't rely on vitamin supplements to make up for a poor diet. Larger amounts of supplements can be toxic. Moreover, certain supplements could backfire and actually increase your cancer risk. Recent research, for example, links beta-carotene supplements with increased risk of both lung and colon cancer. The best advice is to get the maximum amount of vitamins from foods and then to supplement only after reviewing the need with your doctor. Beware of taking megavitamins, especially if you are undergoing treatment. If you take supplements, make sure you take a judicious amount and be sure to clear whatever you're taking with your doctors. Here's why. A study in *Cancer Research* shows that tumors have high nutritional needs. Tumors often "gobble up" mega doses of vitamins so they can grow faster. Until the issue is settled, I'd stay away from megadoses.[5] Following are the supplements that most experts recommend for prostate cancer protection.

Vitamin E: If you are at high risk, you may want to consider taking a daily vitamin E supplement. You'll read about doses of anywhere from 200 IU to 800 IU of vitamin E a day; however, you can obtain this amount only from supplements. If you want to take a vitamin E supplement, consult with your doctor first, since at higher levels vitamin E has been associated with increased risk for bleeding. Your risk of heart disease should be weighed into the equation because vitamin E may be strongly protective against heart disease. I take 400 IU a day.

Vitamin E is one of two supplements that every patient interviewed for this book is taking. The other is selenium.

Selenium: If you want to take a selenium supplement, consult with your physician first. Two hundred micrograms a day is considered safe.

Multivitamin/multimineral: One a day. This is also your easiest and safest source of Vitamin D. Multiminerals may also contain a little selenium.

Lycopene

"Hey, Doc!" A jovial Maine woodsman cornered me at a health fair in the capital city of Augusta. "What about this lycopene stuff? I take a little every day. Is it good for me? I've had prostate cancer and I don't want to get it again." At that point I knew that if lycopene's lore had reached the backwoods of rural New England, it was on its way to becoming a nutritional legend on a par with vitamin C. Lycopene is found in large amounts in tomatoes and gives them their red color. Like vitamin C, lycopene is also an antioxidant, but it may prove much more specific and powerful for prostate cancer protection.

Lycopene hasn't just created a buzz among consumers like my friend from the Maine woods. A groundbreaking study by Omar Kucuk, M.D., and David Wood, M.D., at Wayne State University has doctors talking as well. Here's why. Imagine how hard it is to prove that a supplement or nutrient actually works to protect you against disease. You need to follow thousands of participants over many years. Even then, you'd have a hard time sorting out one nutrient's effects from those of other nutrients. That's why you hear so much conflicting information about so many minerals, vitamins, and supplements. The studies are just plain hard to do. These researchers hit on a brilliant strategy. Why not give lycopene to men who already had prostate cancer and see if it could affect their cancer in the short time between diagnosis and surgery? So the researchers recruited 30 patients whose biopsy results were positive for prostate cancer. One group of patients was given an all-natural tomato lycopene supplement, while another group was given dummy pills so researchers could compare results. Well, the results stunned many doctors.

A key marker for prostate cancer declined by 15 percent in patients taking the lycopene tomato extract. In the control group not taking lycopene, that marker *increased* by 15 percent. When surgeons removed the prostate glands, they found that patients taking lycopene had smaller tumors and that those tumors were more often confined to the prostate. Let's look at the details. In the lycopene-treated group, 73 percent had organ-confined prostate cancer compared to only 18 percent in the control group. Eighty percent had tumors with a volume less than or equal to 4 cubic centimeters in the lycopene group compared to only 45 percent in the control group. This suggested that the group treated with lycopene had tumors that became less malignant. The study also raises a far more interesting and tantalizing, albeit premature, prospect — that the early stages of prostate cancer may be far more easily reversible than had ever been imagined. Although this study gives scientists hope that they can intervene with nutrition to protect men against prostate cancer before it poses a threat to their lives, several scientists, including Dr. Dean Ornish and Dr. Steven Clinton, find the study seriously flawed and believe that Dr. Kucuk's work needs to be repeated.

This study supports the growing body of evidence that lycopene may offer powerful protection against prostate cancer. In fact, ever since Edward Giovannucci, M.D., and his colleagues at Harvard related increased lycopene intake to lower risk of prostate cancer, researchers have been eagerly testing the benefits of lycopene — and have mostly found that lycopene has a protective effect. Now researchers believe that it might even have therapeutic benefits once the disease is diagnosed. This has made lycopene the hottest of media stars. Let's see if it holds up to the limelight.

What Is Lycopene?

In human blood serum, lycopene is the dominant carotenoid and constitutes approximately 50 percent of all carotenoids found in the serum. That's the primer, but here's why researchers have become so intrigued with lycopene's prospects. Lycopene appears in slightly higher concentrations in the prostate. What's more, when you eat lots of tomato-based foods, your blood plasma lycopene levels increase. With increasing age, the lycopene serum values decrease as the risk of prostate cancer increases. This is not to say that one causes the other. Researchers aren't sure whether the drop is because of a biological mechanism related to age or because aging men change their diet to include fewer tomato products. In any case, the irony is that the protective levels of lycopene decrease just as your risk of prostate cancer increases.

Establishing the Link Between Lycopene and Prostate Cancer Protection

Dr. Giovannucci initiated the lycopene–prostate cancer connection. His team examined the dietary lycopene intake of men in the Health Professionals Follow-up Study and found consumption of cooked tomatoes to be linked with a lower risk of prostate cancer. In his study titled "Intake of Carotenoids and Retinol in Relation to Risk of Prostate Cancer," Dr. Giovannucci examined the association between intake of various carotenoids, retinol, and fruits and vegetables and the risk of prostate cancer.[1] He found that lycopene intake *was* associated with a lower risk of prostate cancer. Men who consumed more than 10 servings of tomatoes and tomato products per week had a 35 percent lower risk of prostate cancer than men who ate less than 1.5 servings a week. The three lycopene sources associated with lower prostate cancer risk were, in that order: tomato sauce, tomatoes, and pizza. Tomato sauce, which was the major predictor of higher lycopene blood serum levels, was also the strongest predictor of decreased prostate cancer risk.

How Lycopene Works

Of all the common carotenoids found in the Western diet, lycopene has been shown in test tubes to have the highest oxygen-quenching capacity; in fact, more than double the efficiency of beta-carotene.[2] This oxygen-quenching capacity prevents it from causing DNA havoc. In addition to this antioxidant activity, lycopene's biological activities include growth control and cell-cell communication.

Although researchers do not yet have any recommendations for the actual amount of lycopene that you should ingest, remember that Dr. Giovannucci noted that tomato sauce, tomatoes, and pizza were the primary contributors of lycopene. While lycopene is found in small amounts in a few fruits, tomato products are the richest sources. I have included the table on page 105 so you can make sure you choose foods high in lycopene.

Lycopene Content of Foods

	Serving Size	Weight (grams)	Lycopene (milligrams)
Spaghetti/marinara sauce	½ cup	125	20.0
Tomato sauce	½ cup	123	19.6
Tomato-based vegetable juice	¾ cup	182	17.7
Tomato juice	¾ cup	182	16.9
Tomatoes, canned	½ cup	120	11.6
Tomato puree	¼ cup	63	10.5
Tomato paste	2 tablespoons	33	9.7
Tomato catsup	2 tablespoons	30	5.1
Tomato, raw	1 large (3" diam.)	182	5.5
Tomato, raw	½ cup chopped	90	2.7

Source: USDA–NCC Carotenoid Database for U.S. Foods, 1998.

WHAT YOU CAN DO NOW

Dos and Don'ts of Increasing Your Lycopene Intake

DO include 1 to 2 servings a day of lycopene-rich tomato or tomato products every day for maximum protection. You'll find a wide array of these in food stores.

DO use tomato products that have been heat treated. Lycopene is not well absorbed unless it has been heated — that makes tomato sauce, tomato paste, and catsup the best sources. Be wary of too much sugar and salt in catsup.

DO eat tomato sauces — for example, spaghetti sauce with no red meat.

DO eat whole-wheat pizza with extra tomato sauce but without fatty cheeses and meats.

DO eat cooked tomatoes.

DO buy the reddest tomatoes you can find. Every type of tomato has a slightly different biochemistry, but the redder the tomato the more lycopene it contains.

DO cook tomatoes in a tiny bit of olive oil to help the body absorb lycopene. Lycopene is a highly lipid-soluble chemical, so cooking in a little oil helps release the lycopene antioxidants from tomatoes. Human intestinal absorption of lycopene is also improved in the presence of a little fat or oil. Be careful not to use too much, since you'd be significantly increasing your fat intake, the biggest dietary risk factor for prostate cancer.

DO choose canned tomato juices, since they are all heat treated and also an excellent source of lycopene. One good example is V-8. There are also excellent heat-treated products in bottles such as Knudsen's, which is a brand chosen for a current clinical trial. Steve Clinton, M.D., of the Ohio State University Health Sciences Center emphasizes that most people have enough fat in their meals that if they drink a glass of tomato juice with the meal, the body will be able to absorb the lycopene from the juice.

DON'T eat lycopene-rich foods that are also high in fat — for example fatty spaghetti sauces or white-flour pizza laden with fatty cheeses and meats.

DON'T shy away from fresh tomatoes. They have lots of terrific nutrients. Dr. Clinton concludes that "tomato products of all types are a source of potential cancer-fighting substances. There is nothing wrong with eating tomatoes that are not processed."

The decision to eat more lycopene-containing foods is really a no-brainer. Although we're still awaiting final proof of lycopene's benefit, we do know that lycopene is not harmful and that increasing your intake of tomatoes or tomato products to 1 to 2 servings a day will significantly raise lycopene levels in your blood. Consider them part of the five to nine vegetable and fruit servings recommended by the National Cancer Institute. Since critics are concerned that lycopene is just one of many important antioxidants, the best way to cover yourself is by eating the full nine servings of high-antioxidant fruits and vegetables. You'll find those in the chapter on antioxidants (page 80). For a further critique of lycopene research, see Appendix Two.

Starches and Sugars

During the low-fat revolution, Americans gained, on average, eight pounds. Why? When we gave up fat, many of us replaced fat with starches and sugars instead of fruits, vegetables, and whole grains. What's wrong with too many starches and sugars? The answer is, they force the body to produce large amounts of the hormone insulin, which in turn speeds the storage of fat. New research is investigating high insulin levels in prostate cancer growth. Gail McKeown-Eyssen, Ph.D., epidemiologist at the University of Toronto, says, "Insulin is a growth factor; it may influence the risk of prostate and some other sites of cancer."

How Insulin May Cause Cancer Growth

Test-tube studies have shown that insulin is a growth factor for the prostate cell.[1] Prostate cancer cells have on them specialized receptors. These are the unique locks into which a specialized key must be inserted to turn "on" a certain function, like the lock-and-key principle we looked at for fats. Insulin can turn on these receptors. When there are high levels of either, the cancer may respond to these "growth factors," and, as you would imagine, increase growth.

Elevated insulin levels don't occur in a vacuum. They occur along with elevated levels of blood fats and blood sugar (called glucose), both of which may give the cancer cells lots of extra fuel to grow. Dr. McKeown-Eyssen is now hypothesizing that high insulin levels with the accompanying high glucose levels may be promoting prostate cancer growth in humans. She says: "An increase in glucose may be a source of energy and may increase growth of cancer cells. You're giving cancer cells an optimum environment to grow by giving them both energy and growth factors." What causes a high insulin level? In the short term, it's a response to the dietary excesses we've just looked at, too much starch, too much sugar, and too much fat. In the long term, consistently high insulin levels produce a syndrome called insulin resistance, a state in which individuals have high levels of both insulin and glucose in the blood. They have high glucose levels because the body isn't correctly using insulin to lower glucose levels — that's why it's called insulin *resistance*. Ordinarily, you'd expect that with high insulin levels, blood sugar would be low since insulin's main job is to keep blood-sugar levels from rising. But as insulin becomes ineffective, the body has to make more and more of it and still can't do the job of lowering glucose levels. The results are high levels of insulin, glucose, and blood fats, all potential fuels for increased prostate cancer growth. This syndrome can lead to adult-onset diabetes, and constantly high insulin levels are a fast way to get fat and stay fat. Insulin is the ultimate fat storage hormone.

What's the cause of insulin resistance? There is a certain genetic predisposition, but for insulin resistance to occur, one usually needs to add inactivity, obesity, and the Western diet. The archetypal Western diet is high in fat, high in refined sugars, and low in fruit, fiber, and vegetables; the diet therefore promotes insulin resistance. And insulin resistance — together with its related factors such as high insulin, high glucose, and high blood fats — could promote prostate cancer growth. Insulin resistance can also lead to heart disease, since a blood fat called a triglyceride is elevated while the good cholesterol (HDL) is lowered.

Dr. McKeown-Eyssen is now conducting a study called Insulin Resistance and the Risk of Prostate Cancer. She's measuring blood lipids, blood glucose, insulin, and growth factors in prostate cancer patients to see if they are different from those of individuals who don't have prostate cancer. Her ultimate goal is to find men early in the disease process and then recommend changes in lifestyles such as diet and exercise, which might reduce risk. If there is a final common denominator that ties together all the dangers of the Western lifestyle, it is insulin.

What's Your Insulin Level?

Insulin levels are easy to measure at your annual physical exam; just ask your physician for directions the day before your exam. Your doctor will want to measure your insulin level after an overnight fast, and this measure will be a good indication of whether you may have adult-onset diabetes. A lean person's fasting insulin measures out at less than 5, whereas that of an obese individual can run up to 30. (You can imagine what a difference that much more insulin can make in producing and storing fat.) You can also take a fold of skin right at your belly button. If it's more than one inch, chances are your insulin level is high.

WHAT YOU CAN DO NOW

The best ways to control your insulin are to:

- Cut sugar and starches. Fast-release carbohydrates, like starches, sugars, and refined flours, break down quickly and give rise to elevations in blood-sugar levels. If elevation is sustained during the day by consumption of many of these foods, you have what is called a high glucose load.

The more fast-release carbohydrates you eat in a day, the higher your glucose "load." The Atkins diet, the Sugar Busters! diet, the Suzanne Somers diet, the Dean Ornish diet, and my book *The Revolutionary Weight Control Program* all help you lose weight through the same shared principle — by dropping your glucose load. One or two of these foods a day may not do much harm, but four or more and you are loading up your system with more glucose than it needs, increasing your risk of diabetes and obesity. Dropping these foods entirely is a great way to begin a highly effective weight-loss program. However, eating a high-fat, high-protein diet can increase your risk of prostate cancer and is not recommended here.

On pages 112 and 114 are lists of foods with high and moderate glycemic indexes — you should avoid these. The glycemic index (GI) is a measurement of how much blood sugar rises until it reaches a peak level after a certain food is eaten on an empty stomach. The scale goes from 0 to well over 100.

- Substitute slow-release carbohydrates. Beans, vegetables, many fruits, and high-fiber foods are the carbohydrates you can eat that have the least effect on blood sugar. To help you choose the right carbos, I've included a list of foods with a low glycemic index (page 116).
- Eat whole grains. Grains form the base of the American food pyramid, with up to seven recommended portions per day. What's more, whole grains, as opposed to refined flours, may offer some protection against prostate cancer.

A study from Milan, Italy, showed whole-grain consumption to be associated with a reduced risk of several cancers, including prostate cancer. And a 59-country study showed that grains and cereals are protective against prostate cancer.[2]

High-Glucose Carbohydrates

Food	Glycemic Index
Hamburger bun	61
Ice cream	61
New potato	62
Semolina	64
Shortbread	64
Raisins	64
Macaroni and cheese, boxed	64
Beets	64
Flan	65
Oat kernel	65
Rye flour	65
Couscous	65
High-fiber rye crispbread	65
Sucrose	65
Cream of Wheat (cereal)	66
Life (cereal)	66
Muesli (cereal)	66
Arrowroot	66
Pineapple	66
Angel food cake	67
Croissant	67
Grapenuts (cereal)	67
Puffed wheat (cereal)	67
Breton wheat cracker	67
Stoned Wheat Thins	67
Soft drink, Fanta	68
Cornmeal	68

Food	Glycemic Index
Mars bar	68
Wheat bread, gluten-free	69
Shredded wheat	69
Melba toast	70
Wheat biscuit	70
Potato, white, mashed	70
LifeSavers	70
Fruit, dried	70
Golden Grahams	71
Millet	71
Carrot	71
Bagel, white	72
Water crackers	72
Watermelon	72
Rutabaga	72
Popcorn	72
Kaiser roll	73
Corn chips	73
Honey	73
Bread stuffing	74
Cheerios (cereal)	74
French fries	75
Pumpkin	75
Doughnut	76
Waffle	76
Cocoa Puffs (cereal)	77
Vanilla wafers	77
Broad beans	79
Grapenut Flakes (cereal)	80

Food	Glycemic Index
Jelly beans	80
Puffed crispbread	81
Rice Krispies (cereal)	82
Rice cake	82
Corn Chex (cereal)	83
Potato, instant	83
Cornflakes (cereal)	84
Potato, baked	85
Crispix (cereal)	87
Rice, instant	87
Rice, white, low amylose	88
Rice Chex (cereal)	89
Brown rice pasta	92
French baguette	95
Rockmelon	95
Parsnip	97
Maltose	105
Tofu frozen dessert, nondairy	115

Adapted with permission from *American Journal of Clinical Nutrition* 62: 5, 871S–893S.
Copyright © American Society for Clinical Nutrition.

Moderate-Glucose Carbohydrates

Food	Glycemic Index
Capellini	45
Macaroni, boiled 5 minutes	45
Romano beans	46
Linguine, thick durum	46
Lactose	46

Food	Glycemic Index
Fruit loaf, wheat with dried fruit	47
Instant noodles	47
Bulgur	48
Baked beans	48
Green peas	48
Corn, high amylose	49
Chocolate	49
Rye kernel	50
Ice cream, low fat	50
Tortellini, cheese-filled	50
Yam	51
Kiwifruit	52
Banana	53
Special K (cereal)	54
Buckwheat	54
Sweet potato	54
Potato chips	54
Linseed rye	55
Oatmeal	55
Rich tea biscuit	55
Fruit cocktail, canned	55
Mango	55
Spaghetti, durum	55
Sweet corn	55
Sultanas	56
Potato, white	56
Pita, white	57
Orange juice	57
Bran Chex (cereal)	58

Food	Glycemic Index
Peach, canned, heavy syrup	58
Rice vermicelli	58
Blueberries	59
Pastry	59
Rice, white, high amylose	59
Bran	60
Pizza cheese	60

Adapted with permission from *American Journal of Clinical Nutrition* 62: 5, 871S–89
Copyright © American Society for Clinical Nutrition.

Low-Glucose Carbohydrates

Food	Glycemic Index
Yogurt, low-fat, unsweetened, plain	14
Soybeans	18
Rice bran	19
Cherries	22
Peas, dried	22
Plum	24
Barley	25
Grapefruit	25
Kidney beans	27
Peach, fresh	28
Beans, dried	29
Lentils	29
Green beans	30
Black beans	30
Apricot, dried	31
Butter beans	31
Skim milk	32

Food	Glycemic Index
Lima beans, baby, frozen	32
Split peas, yellow, boiled	32
Chickpeas	33
Rye rice	34
Apple	36
Pear	36
Spaghetti, whole wheat	37
Haricot (navy) beans	38
Star pastina, boiled 5 minutes	38
Tomato	38
Tortilla	38
Brown beans	38
Pinto beans	39
Corn hominy	40
All-Bran	42
Black-eyed peas	42
Grapes	43
Orange	43
Spirali, durum	43
Mixed grain	45

Adapted with permission from *American Journal of Clinical Nutrition* 62: 5, 871S–893S. Copyright © American Society for Clinical Nutrition.

So what are the right grains to eat? The best grains are hunger-cutting grains, grains that reduce your blood-sugar level. These are the most nutritious grains.

The table on page 118 shows how the Washington, D.C.–based Center for Science in the Public Interest (CSPI) ranks grains for their fiber, mineral, and vitamin content.

CSPI Food Values of Grains

Grain (5 oz cooked)	Score
Quinoa	73
Macaroni or spaghetti, whole wheat	69
Amaranth	66
Buckwheat groats	64
Spaghetti, spinach	61
Bulgur	60
Barley, pearled	59
Wild rice	58
Millet	53
Brown rice	51
Triticale	47
Spaghetti	42
Wheat berries	41
Macaroni	39
Kamut	37
Oats, rolled	33
Spelt	33
White rice, converted	26
Couscous	23
White rice, instant	18
Soba noodles	12
Corn grits	10

CSPI came up with a score for each grain by adding its percent of the USRDA for five nutrients (magnesium, vitamin B_6, zinc, copper, and iron) plus fiber. There is no USRDA for fiber so they used the daily value of 25 grams in its place. Copyright © 2000 Center for Science in the Public Interest. Reprinted and adapted from *Nutrition Action Healthletter* (1875 Connecticut Ave. N.W., Suite 300, Washington, D.C. 20009-5728; $24.00 for 10 issues).

The highest score for a grain is 73, whereas the highest ranked vegetable is 461 and the highest ranked bean 300.

Many populations around the world survive and even thrive on a combination of beans and grains. Together these two foods can provide 95 percent of all macro- and micronutrients.

- Cut the animal fat in your diet. Saturated fats change the outer layer of your muscle, called the membrane. A normal muscle membrane lets sugar flow through it easily. Eating large amounts of saturated fats and some polyunsaturated fats makes your muscle far more resistant to the effects of insulin, allowing your blood sugar to rise. Red meat is an animal fat especially high in saturated fats, and studies have repeatedly linked red meat intake and increased risk of prostate cancer.

- Reduce body fat.[3] A study of Seventh-Day Adventists showed that compared with ideal weight, obesity significantly increased the risk of fatal prostate cancer.[4] Men with less-aggressive tumors tend to be leaner than men with highly aggressive tumors. Following the diet guidelines in this book alone will allow you to shed a substantial number of extra pounds of body fat. The men in Dr. Dean Ornish's study lost substantial amounts of weight eating a diet customized for its effect on prostate cancer growth and development. In his earlier cardiac studies, Dr. Ornish found that the patients lost 25 pounds in the first year even though they were eating more food, and more frequently than before (which led to his book *Eat More, Weigh Less*). Adding exercise will speed weight loss. Cutting stress will make weight loss far easier and more pleasurable.

- Eat high-fiber foods. These foods slow the absorption of sugars into the bloodstream. Fiber will also decrease your hunger and keep you feeling full for a longer time. Turn to the fiber chapter for a list of high-fiber foods.

- Exercise has a very powerful effect on decreasing the body's resistance to insulin, so, in turn, insulin levels drop. Turn to the exercise chapter for guidelines (page 202).

Coincidentally, many of the steps used to lower insulin levels are steps you would take to prevent prostate cancer: high fiber, fewer saturated fats, and fewer refined carbohydrates. They're the same steps you'd take to prevent obesity, coronary artery disease, and the risk of adult-onset diabetes.

Note: For men with diabetes, please refer to Appendix Four: A Note for Men with Adult-Onset Diabetes (page 319). A much more detailed explanation of how insulin may increase your risk of cancer through a hormone called Insulin Growth Factor 1 can be found on page 320.

Vitamin D

Lay down a map of the United States. Then plot the numbers of cases of prostate cancer. What will jump out at you is that the farther north you look, the more prostate cancer you'll see. There's actually a gradient from south to north. Simply put, the farther north you live, the higher your risk of prostate cancer. Why? Epidemiologist Gary Schwartz, Ph.D., at the University of Miami in Florida, analyzed the relationship between prostate cancer incidence and the amount of ultraviolet light men are exposed to. Bingo! The graph showed that mortality rates from prostate cancer were highest where ultraviolet exposure was lowest: in the northern parts of the country. And that's not just in America. The highest rates of mortality from prostate cancer in the world are in Scandinavian countries, where annual exposure to ultraviolet light is low.

Why is ultraviolet light so important? The link is to vitamin D. Dr. Schwartz initially observed that patients with higher levels of vitamin D seemed to have lower rates of prostate cancer diagnosed. Ultraviolet light provides the first step in the body's manufacture of vitamin D. Dr. Gary Friedman and colleagues at the Kaiser Health Plan in Oakland, California, also suggest that vitamin D levels might be lower in people who develop prostate cancer. One partial explanation for the increased risk of prostate cancer in black men is that they absorb less ultraviolet light because of their skin pigmentation. So black men who live in northern climates would have an even higher risk due to the limited amount of ultraviolet light and their increased skin pigmentation.

So how does vitamin D affect prostate cells? Prostate cancer cells have vitamin D receptors, report David Feldman, M.D., at Stanford, and Gary Miller, M.D., Ph.D., at the University of Colorado. Think of receptors as on-off switches for cell growth. Dr. Feldman showed that when vitamin D attaches to the vitamin D receptors on prostate cancer cells, the cancer growth slows. He also showed that vitamin D inhibits the growth of noncancerous cells taken from normal prostates of men with an enlarged prostate due to benign prostatic hypertrophy (BPH). In other words, vitamin D is a major brake on prostate growth whether that growth is normal or cancerous.

With that evidence in hand, Dr. Feldman thought, why not test whether vitamin D would slow the growth of prostate cancer in men with the disease? He used the active form of vitamin D, which is called 1,25 dihydroxyvitamin D (nicknamed 1,25-D). And his results provided preliminary evidence that 1,25-D does work, that it is an effective antigrowth agent for prostate cancer! Dr. Feldman studied patients who had a recurrence of their prostate cancer. He followed the cancer growth using a common marker for prostate cancer, measuring how long it would take for the marker to double. Say the marker started out at 2. He would measure how long it took to reach 4. Here's what happened after he gave these patients 1,25-D: the number took up to five times longer to double. In one case, as an example, the doubling time went from 4 months to 20 months! So if the marker started out at 2, rather than reaching 4 in 4 months, it could take nearly 2 years! The full details of the study are found in Appendix Two. You may also want to read Dr. Feldman's excellent book called *Vitamin D,* which clearly explains everything you'll ever want to know about vitamin D.

WHAT YOU CAN DO NOW

Here are the practical and safe measures you can take today:

- Get more sunlight. Since the risk was first identified as too little ultraviolet light, if you live in a northern climate, try to get more exposure to the sun. Solar radiation can provide 75 percent of your daily vitamin D intake. Fortunately, the amount of sun exposure you need for adequate vitamin D synthesis is much less than the amount needed to promote skin cancer. You don't need to stay out long, not long enough to burn, and not when the sun is at its peak intensity — just enough for a healthy glow. Practically speaking, that means getting out into the sun for 15 minutes three times a week.

- Take a daily multivitamin. This has all the vitamin D you need. Dr. Feldman says: "It's important to note that vitamin D supplements are unlikely to be helpful if the patient already takes adequate amounts of vitamin D in the diet." High levels of vitamin D can be toxic. Excessive vitamin D supplements can cause fatally high levels of calcium in the blood. The experts agree: "Although it's too early to give a recommendation of vitamin D for cancer prevention, men should meet the normal daily requirement of vitamin D. That's 200 to 400 international units for adults per day," says Dr. Donald Trump, and Dr. Feldman agrees.

Most ready-to-eat cereals are fortified with 50 IU of vitamin D per ounce.

Calcium

Calcium? A health risk? You've got to be kidding. Drink your milk! How often have you heard that since you were a kid? No doubt about it, calcium makes strong bones. The more calcium you can lay down in your bones, the better long-term hedge you have against osteoporosis. That's just as true for men as it is for women. And that's why it's such a big surprise to most men that excess calcium in the diet could pose a real risk in terms of prostate cancer. That's right. Early scientific studies show an *increased* risk of prostate cancer when you consume large amounts of calcium.

The key study that has scientists and doctors so alarmed is the Health Professionals Follow-up Study. This is a very large and highly respected study conducted out of Harvard University. It showed that when men ingested large amounts of calcium, whether from foods, specific calcium supplements, multivitamins, or even antacids, they increased their risk of prostate cancer. Chief author Dr. Edward Giovannucci noticed that high intake of calcium increased the risk of more aggressive, more advanced, and metastatic or fatal prostate cancer. For men who consumed more than 2,000 milligrams (that's 2 grams) of calcium a day, the risk of advanced cancer was *three* times greater than for men whose calcium intake was less than 500 milligrams a day. To summarize, high calcium intake increased the risk that you would get prostate cancer in the first place *and* the risk that it would be more aggressive *and* the risk that it could become fatal — a triple threat.

June Chan, Sc.D., a research fellow at the Harvard

School of Public Health, also found risks for calcium in a Swedish case control study. She saw a moderately increased risk of prostate cancer associated with higher intake of calcium and dairy products. The men who consumed higher versus lower amounts of calcium and dairy products had an elevated risk of developing more advanced tumors.

What does excess calcium do? We saw in the last chapter how important vitamin D may be to prostate cancer prevention; specifically, the body converts vitamin D into a powerful antitumor hormone called 1,25-D. A high intake of calcium reduces the body's ability to produce 1,25-D. So, in effect, calcium may be reducing the effectiveness of vitamin D.

In this context, switching from drinking cow's milk to soymilk may provide a double benefit (a triple benefit if you believe, as does Dr. T. Colin Campbell, that animal protein, particularly casein, promotes cancer).

As with just about everything in science, not everybody agrees. Dr. Richard Hayes, Ph.D., of the National Cancer Institute, saw in his study no effect of calcium on prostate cancer progression. Many other scientists also contest the Harvard findings. But before you slam the cover of this book in frustration and walk away asking, "Can't scientists ever agree on anything?" read on. You'll find you can take concrete steps right now.

WHAT YOU CAN DO NOW

Consider this. The recommended daily calcium intake (called DRI for Dietary Reference Intake) is 1,000 milligrams for men 19 to 50 years old, and 1,200 milligrams for men 51 years and older. The ironic fact is that many men ingest nowhere near that much, so for them the risk is a moot point. And unless you're drinking over a quart of milk a day, it's impossible to get from your diet the 2,000 milligrams of calcium that was the amount associated with increased risk of advanced disease. In other words, chances are you're well within the safe limits right now.

To clarify the issue further, let's consider these four situations:

- You're at low risk of prostate cancer. Given the limited amount of research, you'd be hard-pressed to make a case for cutting back on calcium intake, especially if you are at risk for osteoporosis.

- You're at high risk of prostate cancer. It's worth having a nutritionist administer a food intake survey to check how much calcium you do ingest. If you're currently taking in more than the recommended intake, discuss with your urologist whether it makes sense to cut back so you are closer to the recommended intake. Since men as well as women are at risk of osteoporosis, you don't want to cheat yourself, either, by eating a lot less than the recommended intake.

- You already have prostate cancer. Consider a lower-calcium diet as a possible means of preventing the cancer from spreading. Avoid supplements containing calcium, including antacids. Look for low-calcium soy protein isolate powders.

- You have advanced prostate cancer. This is a real dilemma. Neil Fleshner, M.D., at the University of Toronto cautions: "I don't recommend my patients go on a low-calcium diet, because we know that hormone treatment of advanced prostate cancers accelerates osteoporosis." Others are concerned that too much calcium could make the cancer worse. Consult with your oncologist to tailor your calcium intake to the requirements of your condition and your current treatment.

Food Sources of Calcium

	Serving Size	Gram Weight	Calcium (mg)
Bread, cereal, rice, pasta			
Bread, whole wheat	1 slice	25	20
Bread, white	1 slice	24	27
Cornflakes	1 cup	28	1
Raisin bran	½ cup	28	20
Pasta, cooked	1 cup	140	24
Rice, brown, cooked	½ cup	97	10
Rice, white, cooked	½ cup	100	8
Vegetables			
Broccoli, cooked	½ cup	78	47
Carrot, raw	1 small	70	13
Corn kernels, cooked	½ cup	82	3
Potato, baked	1 medium	200	12
Tomato, raw	1 medium	123	6
Fruit			
Banana	1 medium	114	7
Berries	½ cup	72	10
Cantaloupe	⅛ melon	150	8
Orange	1 medium	140	52
Meat, fish, poultry, dried beans			
Hamburger, cooked	1 medium patty	100	5
Ham	1 slice	28	2
Chicken breast, skinless	1 medium	86	13

	Serving Size	Gram Weight	Calcium (mg)
Meat, fish, poultry, dried beans, continued			
Halibut, cooked	1 small fillet	85	51
Salmon, cooked	1 small fillet	85	14
Beans, cooked	½ cup	120	80
Lentils, cooked	½ cup	100	19
Tofu, firm	1 oz.	28	58
Eggs			
Whole, boiled	1 large	17	23
Milk, dairy products			
Milk, nonfat	1 cup	24	302
Milk, whole	1 cup	28	148
Cream cheese	2 tablespoons	28	23
Fats, oils			
Insignificant			
Sugar			
Brown sugar	1 teaspoon	5	4
Honey	1 teaspoon	7	0

Source: U.S. Department of Agriculture, Agricultural Research Service, 1999. USDA Nutrient Database for Standard Reference, Release 13.

The table above will give you a good indication of the amount of calcium in foods.

Fiber

Fiber is the most underrated nutrient in our diet today — and that's across the board, whether in the prevention of heart disease, diabetes, cancer, or obesity. Fiber's exceptional powers extend to all these diseases, and that includes prostate cancer. How?

Fiber has the remarkable ability to actually lower plasma levels of the sex hormone testosterone in men eating a diet high in soluble fiber. How does fiber work its wonders? Dr. Neil Fleshner showed that soluble fiber lowered plasma levels of sex hormones by increasing the excretion of these hormones in the men's feces. Dr. Fleshner also followed a prostate cancer marker and found that it dropped by 10 percent after four months on a diet with 18 grams of soluble fiber per day. The key in the study was that the fiber *had* to be soluble fiber, which is found in oats and rice bran; certain vegetables such as Brussels sprouts and carrots; most beans, including soybeans; some fruits such as apples and oranges, and dried fruits. (Soluble fiber interacts with the digestive fluids and sops up water to fill you up. Insoluble fiber — found in foods such as wheat bran, whole grains, and also fruits and vegetables — accelerates the passage of food into the colon, which decreases the amount of time available to digest the food.)

The table on page 130 lists those foods that have the highest content of soluble fiber.

Scientists believe that lowering the levels of hormones such as testosterone could affect the progression of primary

High-Soluble-Fiber Foods

Food	Serving Size	Gram Weight	Soluble Fiber (grams)
Cereals			
Oat bran, generic	½ cup	46	3.5
Oat bran cereal, cold, Quaker	1 cup	37	.9
All-Bran, Kellogg's	½ cup	30	1.5
Oat bran cereal, hot, generic	½ cup	57	2.7
Oatmeal Crisp, General Mills	1 cup	28	1.3
Cheerios, General Mills	1 cup	30	1.3
Complete Oat Bran Flakes, Kellogg's	1 cup	40	1.6
Complete Wheat Bran Flakes, Kellogg's	1 cup	39	1.4
Puffed Wheat, Quaker	1 cup	12	.4
All-Bran with Extra Fiber, Kellogg's	½ cup	28	.9
GrapeNuts, Post	¼ cup	28	.8
Fiber One, General Mills	1 cup	56	1.7
Quaker Oatmeal Squares	1 cup	56	1.6
Nutri-Grain, Kellogg's	1 cup	37	.9
Wheaties, General Mills	1 cup	28	.7
Raisin Bran, Post or Kellogg's	1 cup	52	1.2
Shredded Wheat, Post	1 biscuit	24	.5
Grains			
Rye flour	½ cup	51	2.0
Pearl barley, uncooked	½ cup	100	3.4
Wheat bran	½ cup	30	1.0

Food	Serving Size	Gram Weight	Soluble Fiber (grams)
Grains, continued			
Wheat germ	½ cup	56	1.8
Whole-wheat flour	½ cup	60	1.1
Breads			
Pumpernickel	1 slice	32	1.2
Rye	1 slice	25	.7
Fruits			
Dried apricots	2 halves	7	.3
Dried figs	1 fig	19	.5
Dried prunes	2 prunes	17	.6
Dried peaches	2 halves	26	1.0
Vegetables			
Okra pods, fresh, trimmed	½ cup	50	1.5
Parsley, fresh	¼ cup	15	.4
Brussels sprouts, fresh	½ cup	78	2.0
Turnip, cooked	½ cup	78	1.7
Savoy winter cabbage, fresh	½ cup	35	.7
Legumes (dried, cooked)			
Kidney beans, dark red	1 cup	177	5.7
Cranberry beans	1 cup	177	5.5
Butter beans	1 cup	227	6.6
Black beans	1 cup	172	4.8
Navy beans	1 cup	182	4.4
Pinto beans	1 cup	171	3.8

Reprinted with permission from the HCF Nutrition Research Foundations, Inc.

prostate cancer (we're talking about levels so small that they wouldn't interfere at all with a man's virility). Higher intake of whole-grain foods is related to reduced risk of certain cancers, including prostate cancer,[1] while several studies have shown that low intake of whole-grain cereals is associated with a higher risk of cancer. One of the most important cancer-fighting substances in whole grains is the fiber.[2] Like virtually all the elements discussed in this book, fiber is part of a robust, healthy diet that will help you in several different ways. Says Dr. Fleshner: "I'm a big believer in fiber." Here are some of the additional benefits.

• Weight control. Fiber is critical for controlling hunger and providing the satiation from foods that allows you to control your weight. Fiber slows digestion, thus making food "last longer" and causing your hunger to drop. High-fiber foods are bulkier, have fewer calories, and take longer to eat, which gives your brain a chance to register your food intake before you overeat. The best "anti-hunger" fiber is soluble fiber.

• Heart health. Soluble fiber has been shown to lower modestly cholesterol levels in the blood. Experts believe that fiber directly lowers cholesterol by sucking it into the bowel and excreting it. The Harvard School of Public Health reports that for every additional gram of fiber you eat each day, your risk of heart disease decreases by 2 percent. And for every 2 percent decrease you have in your cholesterol level, there is a 4 percent decrease in your risk of heart disease.

• Control of blood-sugar levels. Fiber holds sugars in the stomach and releases them into the bloodstream very slowly, giving you excellent control over your blood-sugar and insulin levels.

• Other cancers. Whether fiber helps to prevent colon cancer is a matter now of hot debate. A major Harvard study showed it did not. Critics point out that the subjects in this study did not eat large amounts of fiber nor did they eat much soluble fiber, especially that found in bran, so the effect would be hard to see.

WHAT YOU CAN DO NOW

How much fiber? The National Cancer Institute recommends 25 to 35 grams of fiber a day. Dr. Fleshner recommends that one-third of your fiber intake be soluble fiber. Remember that the soluble fiber will also help you control your hunger and weight. The meal plans in this book are engineered to give you 35 grams a day and to provide generous amounts of both soluble and insoluble fiber — so if you're following the menu plans you won't need to worry about soluble versus insoluble since there will be plenty of both! High-fiber cereals and beans offer the most practical way of eating large amounts of soluble fiber.

I'll be the first to admit that for years I turned a blind eye to fiber. Now I make a big effort to get lots of it. To make it simple, I have high-fiber cereal for breakfast and a cup of beans with both lunch and dinner.

Beans are the most fiber-rich foods, but start slowly. A cup of beans rich in soluble fiber can make you uncomfortably full for several hours — the soluble fibers are pulling water into the upper intestine and creating a greater sense of fullness. The other major concern is gas. When you first start eating high-fiber foods, you'll experience an increase in gas — but that should disappear as you become accustomed to eating high-fiber foods. To avoid discomfort, begin by eating no more than half a cup of soluble-fiber foods per day. Increase your ration by one-quarter cup every several days until you reach one and a half cups.

Part Three

Lifestyle

Every morning I roll out of bed and into my study to write. As I begin to collect my thoughts, I say to myself, Wow, this is the way we were meant to live. I think of all the years of bad meals and late nights. Now I simply can't believe how well I feel. It's because of a complete lifestyle I've adapted as part of my prostate cancer protection program. I even think the word *lifestyle* cheapens the concept. How can one feel better or live life more fully? It should be called the lifestyle of kings! The foods and meals sparkle with special nutrients that will make every fiber of your body more alive. The yoga I now practice brings my stress levels to almost zero. And the fitness regime makes me feel like I'm a 25-year-old again. I'm sure you'll feel the same. Sure, you could look at this program as a prescription, but that would be cheating yourself. This is fun! Honest. I just love learning about new and different ways of healing the body while making it stronger and stronger.

What you'll find in this section is the core program with a complete set of meal plans to take you on a real gastronomic adventure, followed by a chapter on stress busting and another on fitness. This part of the book draws together nearly everything anybody knows about prostate cancer protection into a practical and eminently livable plan. It's the plan that millions of men in traditional societies in the Far East have been practicing for centuries. And preliminary studies show that only a combination of these three elements — diet, stress reduction, and exercise — results in a major and measurable decline in the key markers for prostate cancer, even in men who already have the disease. I hope you'll learn to love this lifestyle as much as I have.

If you are a man with prostate cancer, you will want to discuss carefully with your doctor what place lifestyle has in your treatment. Consider this by Dr. Dean Ornish: "If you have *any* treatment for prostate cancer, you may *impede* your sexual function, but following this diet and lifestyle will certainly *improve* your sexual function."

Diet

I love these meals! When they were first designed, I had no idea such great nutrition could have such fabulous taste. I first met their chief architect, Rita Mitchell, R.D., at the *Oprah Winfrey Show* in Chicago. She's a nutritionist from UC Berkeley's Department of Nutrition. Who'd ever believe that a nutritionist could also be a terrific chef! As part of an hour on breast cancer prevention, she had prepared several meals using all of the best ingredients, from soy and broccoli to collards and sweet potatoes. I've got to be honest. I thought, Yuck, this can't possibly taste good. In her big, friendly way, she said, "Go ahead, have a bite." I did and it was like entering a little bit of heaven. Rarely are we treated to new tastes. All of the new aromas and tastes literally exploded in my mouth. Wow! I thought, this is *amazing*. But the real surprise was the aftereffect. Usually after popping some foie gras or a bite of lobster thermidor into your mouth, there's a wonderful mouth feel and great mental "hit." But it fades into a feeling tinged with guilt and heaviness as the effects of the rich, fatty ingredients strike home. After Rita's meal it was, as my kids say, "like, *wow*." There was a level of mental sharpness I've rarely felt. I thought, Gee, is it possible to make great meals that make you feel terrific and are amazingly good for you? Well, Rita and her colleague, Barbara Sutherland, Ph.D., are that fabulous combination of first-rate university nutritionists and great cooks. They can take ingredients that once made many of us shudder to think about and turn them into meals that sing. The genius of Rita and Barbara's meal plans is that they take all the work out of following a prostate cancer protection program. Without them, you'd feel like a chemist, trying to mix enough lycopene, genistein, selenium, and other ingredients into your foods. This way, it's all done for you, sort of like a nutritional autopilot. Rita and Barbara have meticulously incorporated each of these ingredients into really great meals.

All of the meal plans and recipes in this chapter were developed by Rita Mitchell, R.D., and Dr. Barbara Sutherland of the University of California, Berkeley, at my request, to meet the recommendations in this book. I've cooked these simple-to-prepare dishes myself. They're quick, with just a few steps. I've included the recipes for some of the meals that you may be unfamiliar with. My forthcoming cancer-fighting cookbook, however, will contain the recipes for *all* the meals mentioned in this chapter. For other recipe ideas, I strongly recommend Michael Milken's two books, *The Taste for Living Cookbook* and *The Taste for Living WORLD Cookbook*. Mike has taken the next step in meal design by engineering meals that look and taste like popular American foods but incorporate all the key strategies of prostate cancer protection. Dean Ornish's books, *Eat More, Weigh Less, Everyday Cooking with Dr. Dean Ornish,* and *Dr. Dean Ornish's Program for Reversing Heart Disease,* have many excellent low-fat recipes as well. In his clinical trial, in which he is treating prostate cancer patients with nutrition, Dean uses diets very similar to those you'll find in his books. Depending on how aggressive your prostate cancer protection plan is, you may have to make minor modifications to his recipes, such as restricting dairy to reduce calcium intake.

K. Dun Gifford, president and founder of Oldways Preservation Trust, the country's premier food issues think tank, promotes healthy eating based on traditional foodways.

His organization chooses diets based on three criteria. The first is nutritional science, which considers these elements: epidemiological studies such as those showing that men in China and Japan have lower prostate cancer rates; laboratory analyses of foods to measure antioxidant properties, saturated fat content, et cetera; and dietary intervention trials that hire people to adopt these diets for a few months or years in order to examine changes in blood serum such as cholesterol.

The second criterion for choosing diets is familiarity and accessibility of foods. People don't change their dietary habits with strange foods. Luckily, the world's healthiest diets contain foods that are extremely palatable, familiar, and fun to us — Italian and Greek, Chinese and Japanese food.

The third criterion is whether there is a strong cultural tradition of some durability behind these diets. The traditional diets you'll find in this book are two thoroughly studied by Oldways: the Mediterranean and Asian diets. Both have been around for millennia. They offer an excellent balance of nutrients and contain whole rather than processed grains. You'll also find a New American plan that uses foods much closer to home.

Let's take a look. First, you should know that:

- The diets in all three menus contain 40 grams of soy protein — 20 grams from meals and 20 grams from a shake. So, whatever menu you choose, remember to add one soy shake to your diet per day.

SOY PROTEIN SHAKE RECIPE

This shake provides 20 grams of soy protein. It is an excellent, nutritious afternoon "pick-me-up." If you like, have half a recipe for a mid-morning or nighttime snack, and the other half for an afternoon snack.

You may substitute other fruits for the banana and strawberries. For a thicker shake, freeze the fruit ahead of time.

Yield: 1 serving

1 cup nonfat soy drink
2 tablespoons packed soy protein powder
1 tablespoon orange juice concentrate
½ medium banana, cut in chunks
½ cup strawberries

Put all ingredients in a blender. Blend until smooth.

- You'll want to add to your meals one 6-ounce glass of canned tomato juice a day. Make sure you drink this glass with a meal to enable maximum lycopene absorption.
- All of the menus meet all of the dietary recommendations in Part II of this book.
- All of the meal plans have 800 milligrams of calcium, which is a little less than the daily requirement. If you and your doctor feel you need more calcium, you may want to consider some of the sources in the calcium chapter rather than supplements or calcium contained in antacids.

Asian Menus

These are the premier prostate cancer protection meals. The World Health Organization (WHO) is the premier arbiter of how a country fails or succeeds in preventing illness. The WHO reports that between 1990 and 1993 there were 17.5 prostate cancer deaths per 100,000 men in the United States, whereas in Japan the rate was only 4 deaths per 100,000 men. The low-fat, high-fruit, high-vegetable, and soy-based diet may be the most important reason for the differing rates. Consistently, of all the world's healthy diets, the ones that are the most prostate healthy come from the Far East. The menus below contain whole grains and at least 9 servings of fruits and vegetables a day, including two cruciferous vegetables and one serving of lycopene-rich tomato products. The meals are low in fat (10 percent of total calories), have *no* dairy or other animal products, and have approximately 35 grams of total dietary fiber a day. They provide about 20 grams of soy protein from the menu items. Remember to make one soy protein shake a day and to drink one 6-ounce glass of canned tomato juice with a meal every day. If you're at high risk or have prostate cancer, these are the meals I recommend most strongly because they mirror the foods eaten by men in the Far East.

BREAKFAST

Soy Breakfast Smoothie

(Nonfat soymilk, banana, orange juice, and soy protein powder with vanilla and nutmeg flavoring)

Rice and Vegetables

Tempeh with Snow Peas, Mushrooms, and Carrots

(Vegetables and soy tempeh seasoned with hoisin sauce, mirin, and fresh ginger, served over brown rice)

Apple and Pear Slices

Vegetable Pho

(Flavorful spicy broth with rice noodles, fresh green soybeans, tomatoes, green onions, bean sprouts, and cilantro)

Sliced Orange

Griddle Rice Cakes with Curried Tofu

(Brown and short-grain rice cakes served with a curry of onions, bell peppers, and tofu and topped with cilantro)

Fresh Papaya and Mango Chutney

Miso Soup

(Miso-flavored broth with carrots, shiitake mushrooms, slivered tofu, green onions, and brown rice)

Fresh Cherries and Mandarin Orange Slices

LUNCH

Tofu Mushroom Soup

(Julienne strips of firm tofu, black mushrooms, button mushrooms, shiitake mushrooms, bok choy, and leeks in vegetable broth seasoned lightly with miso and oyster sauce)

Mixed-Vegetable Stir-Fry

Orange Slices in Orange Water

Mu Shu Vegetables

(Bean sprouts, black mushrooms, shredded carrots, bok choy, onions, and cabbage, wrapped in mu shu wrappers and garnished with plum sauce and chopped green onions)

Carrot Daikon Salad

Asian Pear and Apple Slices

Broccoli-Mushroom Stir-Fry with Tofu

(Broccoli florets, shiitake mushrooms, snow peas, water chestnuts, green onions, and tofu in a stir-fry seasoned with chili and fresh ginger, served over brown rice)

Watercress Salad

Kiwi Fruit and Pear Slices

Sweet and Sour Tofu

(Pineapple chunks, sweet red peppers, broccoli florets, large pieces of onion, and tofu in a sweet and sour sauce, served over brown rice)

Asparagus and Radish Salad

Mandarin Orange Wedges

Vegetables and Tofu with Noodles

(Richly seasoned stir-fried broccoli, cauliflower, bok choy, black mushrooms, sweet red peppers, onions, water chestnuts, and tofu, served over rice noodles and garnished with cilantro)

Bean Sprout Salad

Banana and Dried Cranberries

DINNER

Cauliflower and Carrot Curry with Tofu

(Tofu with tomatoes, carrots, onions, cauliflower, and green beans, in a curry of garlic, ginger, turmeric, coriander, and cumin, served over brown rice)

Mint Chutney

Lychees and Mango Ice

Laotian Soup

(Fresh green soybeans, green onions, tomatoes, carrots, and broccoli in a vegetable broth flavored with lemongrass, roasted garlic, hoisin sauce, and cilantro, served over brown rice)

Pickled Cucumbers and Onions

Banana Baked in Orange Water

Sweet and Sour Bok Choy and Tempeh

(Soy tempeh with bok choy, carrots, green peppers, red onion, pineapple chunks, and ginger in a tangy sweet and sour sauce, served over brown rice)

Vietnamese Salad Rolls

Mango Sorbet

Grilled Tofu and Tomato

Fresh Vegetable Medley

(Onions, broccoli, cauliflower, snow peas, sweet red peppers, and fresh green soybeans in a light sauce flavored with chili)

Papaya and Strawberries

Rice Noodles with Vegetables and Tofu in Black Bean Sauce

(A stir-fry of firm tofu, green beans, onions, bok choy, broccoli, shiitake mushrooms, carrots, and sweet red peppers in black bean sauce, served over rice noodles)

Bean Sprout Salad

Mung Bean Cake

RECIPES FOR THE ASIAN MENUS

VEGETABLE PHO

Yield: 2 servings

Preparation time: 15 minutes

Cooking time: 25 minutes

Ingredients

4 cups vegetable stock, homemade or canned

3 cloves roasted garlic, minced

1 teaspoon grated fresh ginger

1-inch piece lemongrass, smashed using the side of a knife

1-inch length cinnamon stick

¼ teaspoon fish sauce

¼ teaspoon tamari soy sauce

¼ teaspoon red pepper flakes

¼ teaspoon sugar

4 ounces pho rice noodles

1 medium tomato, chopped

1 medium green onion cut in 1-inch pieces and sliced thinly
   lengthwise
½ cup fresh green soybeans
1 cup mung bean sprouts, rinsed
6 sprigs cilantro, leaves only

1. In a large saucepan, combine stock, garlic, ginger, lemongrass, cinnamon, fish sauce, soy sauce, pepper flakes, and sugar. Bring to a boil, reduce heat, cover, and simmer gently for 20 minutes.

2. Meanwhile, boil four quarts of water in a large saucepan. Remove from heat, add noodles, and let stand 10– 15 minutes until noodles are tender, stirring occasionally. Drain.

3. Strain broth to remove the solid bits. Return broth to pan. Add tomato, green onion, and soybeans. Heat for 5 minutes.

4. Put noodles into serving bowls. Top with mung bean sprouts. Ladle broth and vegetables into the bowls.

5. Top with cilantro.

BROCCOLI-MUSHROOM STIR-FRY WITH TOFU

Yield: 2 servings

Preparation time: 10 minutes

Cooking time: 15 minutes

Ingredients

¼ teaspoon canola oil
1 cup broccoli florets (grape-size pieces)
2 cloves roasted garlic, minced
18 snow peas
4 small shiitake mushrooms, chopped

4 medium green onions, chopped
½ cup sliced water chestnuts
6 drops chili oil
6 drops tamari soy sauce
1 teaspoon sherry vinegar
1 teaspoon grated fresh ginger
4 ounces firm tofu, in irregular-shaped pieces
2 cups cooked brown rice

1. In a large skillet or wok, heat oil over medium heat. Add broccoli and garlic; cook about 5 minutes, stirring constantly.

2. Add snow peas, mushrooms, green onions, and water chestnuts. Cook about 5 minutes longer, stirring constantly.

3. Add chili oil, soy sauce, sherry vinegar, and ginger; gently mix into vegetables.

4. Add tofu. Stir gently. Continue cooking 2–3 minutes, just to heat tofu.

5. Serve over brown rice.

CAULIFLOWER AND CARROT CURRY WITH TOFU

Yield: 2 servings

Preparation time: 15 minutes

Cooking time: 15 minutes

Ingredients

2 tablespoons cornstarch
1¾ cup water
½ teaspoon canola oil
¼ medium onion, chopped
2 cloves roasted garlic, minced
½ tablespoon grated fresh ginger

1 teaspoon cumin powder
1 teaspoon dried coriander leaf
⅛ teaspoon turmeric
1 cup small cauliflower florets
1 small carrot, thinly sliced
1 cup sliced green beans
1 small tomato, chopped
4 ounces extra-firm tofu, cubed
2 cups cooked brown rice
1 tablespoon chopped fresh cilantro

1. In a small bowl, mix cornstarch with ¼ cup water to a smooth paste. Add remaining water, stir to combine. Set aside.

2. In a medium skillet or wok, heat canola oil over medium-high heat. Add onion and garlic. Cook for 3 minutes.

3. Stir in ginger, cumin, coriander, and turmeric. Add cauliflower, carrot, and green beans. Cook for 4 minutes.

4. Gently stir in tomato and cook for 3 minutes to heat tomato.

5. Pour cornstarch mixture over the vegetables. Bring to a boil, stirring constantly.

6. Add tofu, stir gently, and cook for 1 minute to warm the tofu.

7. Serve over rice and garnish with fresh cilantro.

FRESH VEGETABLE MEDLEY

Yield: 2 servings
Preparation time: 15 minutes
Cooking time: 15 minutes

Ingredients

 ½ tablespoon cornstarch

 ¼ cup cold water

 4 drops chili oil

 1 teaspoon canola oil

 ¼ cup chopped onion

 ½ cup small broccoli florets

 ½ cup small cauliflower florets

 ½ cup diagonally sliced snow peas

 ¾ cup fresh green soybeans

 ¼ medium sweet red pepper, cut in ½-inch pieces

 ¼ cup sliced water chestnuts

 8 medium cherry tomatoes

 2 cups cooked brown rice

1. In a small bowl, mix cornstarch with water to a smooth paste. Add chili oil. Stir and set aside.

2. In a medium skillet or wok, heat canola oil over medium-high heat. Add onion and cook for 3 minutes.

3. Add broccoli, cauliflower, snow peas, and soybeans. Cook for 3 minutes longer.

4. Add red pepper and water chestnuts. Cook for 2 minutes.

5. Pour cornstarch mixture over the vegetables. Bring to a boil, stirring constantly. Add cherry tomatoes and stir gently.

6. Serve over brown rice.

New American Menus

If you say, "Okay, Dr. Bob, you've taken your best shot, but there's no way you're going to find me eating all these exotic foreign foods," these meal plans are for you. They are simple American meals that incorporate all that we've learned in the last section of the book. The New American menus contain 9 servings of fruits of fruits and vegetables a day, including two cruciferous vegetables and one serving of lycopene-rich tomato products. They are low in fat (10% of the total calories from fat), high in total dietary fiber (approximately 35 grams a day) and provide approximately 20 grams of soy protein a day from the menus. They contain no animal products. You'll want to add a soy protein shake to your diet every day (see recipe on page 142). You'll also want to add one 6-ounce glass of canned tomato juice with a meal every day. These meals, too, are designed for men at high risk for prostate cancer. One final point. The experience of low-fat nutrition pioneer Nathan Pritikin and others has been that even if you choose the most stringent diet, you may find that while you aim at eating a 10 percent fat diet, you may end up closer to 15 or even 20 percent. For that reason, you may want to consider a stricter program, realizing that you could end up eating more fat anyhow.

BREAKFAST

Homemade Muesli
(A mixture of rolled oats, wheat flakes, soy protein powder, oat bran, and dried apricots)
Orange Slices
Grapefruit Juice

Steel-Cut Oatmeal with Sun-Dried Cranberries
Orange Juice

Baked Tofu Florentine
(Savory baked tofu served over wilted spinach, coated with a low-fat sauce, and dusted with toasted whole wheat breadcrumbs)

Seven-Grain Bread
Apple-Cranberry Juice

Buckwheat Pancakes with Berries
(Dense, grainy, buckwheat pancakes laden with fresh berries)
Mango-Guava Nectar

All-Bran Cereal with Soy Drink and Banana-Pineapple Juice

LUNCH

Vegetable-Potato Salad
*(Carrots, asparagus, potatoes, shredded red cabbage, Fuji apple, red
onion, and parsley, lightly dressed with balsamic vinegar and a
drop of olive oil, served on a bed of baby bok choy leaves)*
Sesame Seed Roll
Kiwi Fruit

Bean and Broccoli Burrito with Tomato-Corn Salsa
*(Whole wheat tortilla filled with black beans, brown rice, broccoli florets,
and green onions, served with fresh tomato-corn salsa and cilantro)*
Strawberry and Orange Fruit Plate

Kale and Cucumber Soup
*(A creamy soup of kale, cucumbers, and green onions,
seasoned with roasted garlic and dill)*
Whole Wheat Bran Roll
Lemon-Raspberry Sorbet

Open-Face Lentil-Loaf Sandwich
*(Lentil loaf topped with sun-dried tomatoes and a sprinkle of chopped
green onions served warm on a whole-wheat baguette)*
Fresh Spinach and Red Cabbage Salad
Dried Fig Slices

Spring Artichoke Heart Salad

(Baby artichoke hearts, sweet red peppers, cauliflower, mushrooms, green peas, lightly dressed with balsamic vinegar and a drop of olive oil, served over brown rice)

Low-Fat Whole Wheat Crackers

Mandarin Orange Wedges

DINNER

Black Bean and Mushroom Stew with Parsley Polenta

(Shiitake and button mushrooms with black beans in a tomato-vegetable broth served with parsley polenta)

Steamed Broccoli

Garden Salad

Peach Slices and Raspberries with Lemon Sorbet

Grilled Tofu with Roasted Corn and Red Pepper Salsa

Quinoa

Lemon Carrots and Collard Greens

Crusty Dinner Roll

Ginger Silken Tofu

Three Bean Chili

(Spicy chili made with three beans [soybeans, black beans, and Christmas lima beans], onions, celery, kale, and green chilies in a tomato-vegetable broth)

Warmed Whole Wheat Tortillas

Mixed Greens and Tomato

Honeydew Melon and Blueberries

Black Bean and Rice Soup

(A hearty soup of black beans, brown rice, vegetables, and tempeh)

Crusty French Bread

Spinach and Orange Salad

Fresh Figs and Persian Melon Slices

Stuffed Red Peppers

(Large red peppers stuffed with brown rice, wild rice, broccoli florets, black beans, green onions, and raisins, with tomato sauce, topped with toasted whole wheat bread crumbs)

Steamed Fresh Asparagus

Grainy Whole Wheat Roll

Baked Apple

RECIPES FOR THE NEW AMERICAN MENUS

HOMEMADE MUESLI

Because Muesli stores well, we also give ingredient quantities for 16 servings. Store the combined dry ingredients in an airtight container in a cool, dry place for a quick and easy workday breakfast.

Yield: 2 servings, ½ cup each

Preparation time: 10 minutes

Cooking time: None

Ingredients

2 servings	16 servings *to make ahead*	
½ cup	4 cups	rolled oats
¼ cup	2 cups	wheat flakes
2 tablespoons	1 cup	packed soy protein powder
1 tablespoon	½ cup	oat bran
4 halves	32 halves	dried apricots, chopped
¼ cup		nonfat soymilk

1. Combine all dry ingredients.
2. Serve ½ cup in each bowl.
3. Add soymilk.

BEAN AND BROCCOLI BURRITO WITH TOMATO-CORN SALSA

Yield: 2 servings, 1 burrito each
Preparation time: 30 minutes
Cooking time: None

Ingredients

¼ teaspoon canola oil
⅔ cup broccoli florets (grape-size pieces)
4 medium green onions, chopped
⅔ cup cooked brown rice
⅔ cup canned black beans, drained, not rinsed
½ cup chopped tomato
¼ cup white corn, fresh or frozen
2 tablespoons chopped cilantro
2 ten-inch flour tortillas
sprinkle red chili powder, if desired

1. Heat oil over medium heat in a nonstick pan. Add broccoli and green onion. Stir constantly, about 3–5 minutes, until vegetables are soft.

2. Add brown rice and black beans. Cook until mixture is hot, stirring gently.

3. Make salsa by mixing tomato, corn, and cilantro in a small bowl.

4. Soften tortillas by placing in a hot skillet for a few seconds.

5. Spread rice and bean mixture along center of tortilla. Top with salsa. Add chili powder if desired.

6. Fold opposite sides of tortilla over about 1 inch of filling, then roll the tortilla over the filling.

GRILLED TOFU WITH ROASTED CORN
AND RED PEPPER SALSA

Yield: 2 servings

Preparation time: 25 minutes

Cooking time: 10 minutes

Ingredients

1 ear corn

½ medium sweet red pepper

2 three-ounce portions savory baked tofu

½ cup chopped tomato

1½ teaspoons chopped cilantro

⅛ teaspoon salt

Preheat oven to 400 degrees F.

1. Remove husks and silk from corn. Rinse corn and cut kernels from cob. Place on foil-lined cookie sheet.

2. Remove stem, seeds, and membranes from pepper. Rinse pepper; place on cookie sheet with corn.

3. Roast corn and pepper in oven for 15 minutes. Remove from oven; let cool. Preheat broiler.

4. Place tofu on grilling rack; broil for 2–3 minutes on each side.

5. Meanwhile, peel loose skin from pepper; dice finely. Combine pepper, corn, tomato, cilantro, and salt. Stir lightly to mix.

6. Serve tofu topped with salsa.

THREE BEAN CHILI

Yield: 6 servings

Preparation time: 20 minutes

Cooking time: 15 minutes

Ingredients

1 teaspoon olive oil

1 medium onion, chopped

2 cups cooked Christmas lima beans

15-ounce can black beans, drained, not rinsed

15-ounce can soybeans, drained, not rinsed, or 2 cups cooked
mature soybeans

1 medium turnip, cubed

2 stalks celery, coarsely chopped

2 cups vegetable stock

1½ cups tomato juice

3½-ounce can diced green chilies

1 teaspoon red chili powder

1 teaspoon cumin powder

1. In a large pot, heat olive oil over medium-high heat. Add onion, cook for 15 minutes until onion is deep golden.

2. Add all other ingredients, stir gently.

3. Bring to a boil. Reduce heat and simmer for 10–15 minutes until vegetables are soft.

Mediterranean Menus

The Mediterranean meal plan is for men who are at lower risk or do not want to undertake the strictest regimen (but may not go far enough if you have prostate cancer or are at risk for it). The ingredients are readily available in supermarkets. Mediterranean men have far less prostate cancer and heart disease than American men, but not as low rates as men in the Far East. The menus contain at least 9 servings of fruits and vegetables a day, including two cruciferous vegetables and one serving of lycopene-rich tomato products. They are moderate in fat, containing 15 to 20 percent of the calories from fat, mostly olive oil. Because of the inclusion of whole grains, fruits, vegetables and legumes, they are high in total dietary fiber. They contain about 20 grams of soy protein from menu items. You'll have to add a soy protein shake to your diet every day (see recipe on page 141). Be sure, too, to drink a 6-ounce glass of canned tomato juice with at least one meal every day.

BREAKFAST

Goat Cheese with Melon and Figs
Toasted Dense Whole Wheat Bread
Orange Juice

Artichoke Frittata
(Low-fat frittata made with artichoke hearts, green and red peppers, and savory baked tofu)
Baked Roma Tomato with Fresh Basil
Black Olive Focaccia
Grapefruit Juice

Cornmeal Waffles with Peaches and Berries
(Crispy waffles made of whole wheat flour, cornmeal, and soy protein powder)
Pineapple Juice

Buckwheat Crepes with Date-Orange Filling

(Buckwheat and whole wheat flour crepes filled with oranges and dates, topped with nonfat yogurt flavored with orange juice)

Strawberry-Guava Nectar

Breakfast Smoothie

(Sliced peaches, yogurt, orange juice concentrate, and vanilla soymilk)

Toasted Whole Wheat Nut Bread

LUNCH

Pita Bread Sandwich

(A whole wheat pita bread filled with soybean hummus, sweet red peppers, and shredded cabbage, topped with chopped black olives, Italian parsley, and nonfat plain yogurt)

Roma Tomatoes with Olive Oil

Fuji Apple Slices and Figs

Minestrone

(A hearty mixture of potatoes, carrots, celery, cabbage, French beans, rutabaga, and collard greens, with garbanzo beans, kidney beans, and fresh green soybeans in a tomato-vegetable broth)

Whole Wheat Focaccia

Bosc Pear Slices

Spring Cracked Wheat Salad

(Asparagus, mushrooms, red cabbage, green onions, and walnuts, dressed lightly and served on a bed of cracked wheat mixed with cooked soybeans, sprinkled with low-fat feta cheese)

Crisp Breadsticks

Sliced Kiwi Fruit and Banana

Greek Sandwich

(Crusty roll filled with pears, walnuts, and a creamy blend of silken tofu and soy protein powder with romaine lettuce and crumbled low-fat feta cheese)

Broccoli Salad

Strawberries

Roasted Pepper and Eggplant Salad

(Eggplant, red, yellow, and green sweet peppers, zucchini, green onions, and cauliflower, lightly tossed in a yogurt–garlic dressing, garnished with raisins)

Flatbread with Soybean Hummus

Plums

DINNER

Vegetable and Bean Ragout over Couscous

(Garbanzo beans, soybeans, sweet red peppers, onions, turnips, and kale, seasoned with coriander, cinnamon, cardamom, and turmeric, served over couscous)

Field Greens

Apple and Grapefruit Slices with Currants

Green Cabbage Stuffed with Bulgur and Vegetables

(Cabbage leaves stuffed with bulgur, mushrooms, butternut squash, soybeans, onions, raisins, sunflower seeds, and dried figs, seasoned with nutmeg and cumin)

Baked Roma Tomato with Fresh Basil

Whole Wheat Roll

Fresh Strawberries with Lemon Sorbet

Bouillabaisse

(Variety of fresh fish with leeks, celery, tomatoes, sweet red peppers, rutabaga, and broccoli in a rich broth seasoned with garlic, basil, saffron, and orange peel)

French Bread

Romaine Lettuce with Balsamic Vinegar Dressing

Mixed Berry Ice

Ratatouille

(A robust casserole of eggplants, onions, green peppers, zucchini, tomatoes, rutabagas, and fresh green soybeans, seasoned with basil and oregano)

Soft Breadsticks

Spinach and Orange Salad

Minted Melon Slices

Linguine with Lentils

(A flavorful tomato sauce with collard greens, lentils, and soy tempeh served over linguine, dusted with freshly grated Parmesan cheese)

Steamed French Green Beans

Hearty Bread

Plums with Yogurt

RECIPES FOR THE MEDITERRANEAN MENUS

CORNMEAL WAFFLES WITH PEACHES AND BERRIES

Yield: 2 servings

Preparation time: 20 minutes

Cooking time: 20 minutes

Ingredients

1 large peach, sliced

1 cup blueberries

½ cup whole wheat flour

¼ cup cornmeal

2 tablespoons packed soy powder

pinch salt
2 teaspoons baking powder
1 tablespoon brown sugar
1 large egg, separated
1 cup nonfat soymilk

Preheat waffle iron according to manufacturer's instructions.

1. Combine peach and blueberries in a small bowl. Set aside.

2. Stir together flour, cornmeal, soy powder, salt, baking powder, and sugar in a medium bowl.

3. In a small bowl, beat egg yolk; add soymilk and mix until blended.

4. In another bowl, beat egg white until it forms soft peaks when the blade is lifted.

5. Make a well in the dry ingredients; pour egg and soy mixture into the flour mixture. Stir gently to combine.

6. Gently fold in the beaten egg whites. Do not beat.

7. Bake in preheated waffle iron according to manufacturer's directions.

8. Top with fruit.

PITA BREAD SANDWICH

Yield: 2 servings

Preparation time: 10 minutes

Cooking time: None

Ingredients

2 pita breads per serving
½ cup Soybean Hummus (recipe follows)
½ cup chopped sweet red pepper

1 cup shredded green cabbage

½ cup chopped tomato

¼ cup plain nonfat yogurt

2 tablespoons sliced black olives

2 tablespoons chopped Italian parsley

1. Cut pita bread in half, or cut a small section from one edge to make a pocket.

2. Spread hummus on the inside bottom part of the pita. Fill the pita pocket with red pepper, cabbage, and tomato.

3. Spread yogurt on top. Sprinkle evenly with olives and parsley.

SOYBEAN HUMMUS

Yield: 1 cup

Preparation time: 5 minutes

Cooking: None

Ingredients

1 cup cooked mature soybeans or canned soybeans

1 teaspoon tahini

5 teaspoons lemon juice

1 tablespoon olive oil

4 drops sesame oil

2 tablespoons water

⅛ teaspoon cayenne

1. Put all ingredients in a blender.

2. Process until smooth.

MINESTRONE

Yield: 6 servings

Preparation time: 30 minutes

Cooking time: 1 hour total

Ingredients

2 tablespoons olive oil

½ medium onion, chopped

2 stalks celery with leaves, chopped

2 cloves roasted garlic, minced

1 medium potato, scrubbed and diced

1 medium rutabaga, peeled and diced

1 large carrot, peeled and diced

4 cups vegetable stock, homemade or canned

4 cups tomato juice

2 tablespoons tomato paste

1 cup French beans, trimmed and cut in half

1 cup chopped collard greens

1 cup shredded cabbage

1 cup uncooked large pasta shells

15-ounce can garbanzo beans, drained, not rinsed

15-ounce can red kidney beans, drained, not rinsed

2 cups fresh green soybeans

½ teaspoon salt

¼ teaspoon pepper

H teaspoon oregano

1. Heat olive oil in a large, heavy saucepan.

2. Add onion, celery, and garlic; sauté for about 5 minutes until vegetables are lightly browned.

3. Add potato, rutabaga, and carrot; continue cooking for an additional 5 minutes.

4. Add stock, tomato juice, and tomato paste; bring to a boil.

5. Add French beans, collard greens, and cabbage.

6. When soup returns to boil, add pasta. Simmer for 20 minutes.

7. Add beans and seasonings. Cook for 2 minutes longer.

LINGUINE WITH LENTILS

Yield: 2 servings

Preparation time: 15 minutes

Cooking time: 25 minutes

Ingredients

4 teaspoons olive oil

½ medium onion, chopped

2 cloves roasted garlic, minced

1 cup tomato sauce

¾ cup vegetable stock, homemade or canned

¼ teaspoon oregano

¼ teaspoon basil

¼ teaspoon salt

⅛ teaspoon pepper

½ cup cooked lentils

4 ounces soy tempeh, crumbled

3 cups shredded collard greens

4 ounces linguine

1 tablespoon grated Parmesan cheese

1. Heat olive oil over medium heat in a nonstick saucepan.

2. Add onions and garlic and sauté for 5 minutes until soft.

3. Add tomato sauce, vegetable stock, seasonings, lentils, and tempeh.

4. Bring to boil, reduce heat, and simmer for 10 minutes.

5. In another saucepan, steam the collard greens for 10 minutes; add to sauce. Stir to mix well.

6. Meanwhile, bring 4 quarts of water to a boil. Add ⅛ teaspoon salt and a few drops of olive oil.

7. Add linguine noodles; cook for 15 minutes until tender. Drain but do not rinse.

8. Put noodles onto plates or pasta bowls, top with sauce, and sprinkle with Parmesan cheese.

Supplements

To the Asian, New American, and Mediterranean meal plans you can add a few very basic supplements after consulting with your doctor:

- 200 to 800 IU vitamin E
- 200 micrograms selenium
- Multivitamin low in calcium but containing 200 to 400 IU of vitamin D

Eating Out

"When possible, choose restaurants that prepare foods in a way to meet your health needs. The time and effort it takes to locate a few restaurants/cafes that prepare your type of food are well worth it." That's what I originally wrote to open this section. And I mean it! But I'm sure you're saying, "Sure! Dr. Bob, I'll just tell my best client we're going to the Tofu Bar! Or let my wife know that our anniversary is going to be at the local vegan restaurant, or tell my 6-year-old that his birthday party is at the health bar. That'll really go over well!" I hope in the future that healthier restaurants *will* go over better with clients and family. But until they do, here's what to look for in the hard-bitten world of commercial dining! Remember, when you become a regular customer, the chef and wait staff will be more eager to accommodate your needs.

Full-Service Restaurants

Full-service restaurants where food is prepared on site are your best bet. Because foods are prepared to order, the chef can make modifications in preparing your particular meal. There are certain foods that restaurants always stock. You can always request extra fresh vegetables, for instance, or broiled tomato to accompany your meal. Ask for lots of fresh chopped parsley to sprinkle on top instead of Parmesan cheese. Choose broth-based vegetable soups over cream soups or hearty meat soups. Select items without batter or crumbs that are grilled, broiled, poached, or baked. Request that foods be prepared without sauces. Ask that salad dressing be served on the side, and use vinegar and a small amount of olive oil.

And even if it's not on the menu, you can always ask for a plate of steamed vegetables without any added oil or butter. You don't have to make a big deal about it or draw attention to yourself — and you may find that your meal looks better than everyone else's!

Delis and Take-Out-Service Counters

Delis are becoming more responsive to the needs of people wanting to make healthy choices. Pilafs and salads made from beans or lentils or from bulgur, brown rice, and other whole grains are becoming more available. Have the server drain as much of the dressing as possible. Sandwiches with roasted vegetables or lettuce, tomatoes, and cucumber slices can be ordered on whole-grain bread. Spicy mustard is great; hold the mayo. Whole fresh fruit or cut-up fruit salads are usually available. If not, ask for them.

Juice Bars

Juice bars usually offer made-to-order smoothies or blended fruit drinks. Most of them will fit nicely into your meal plan because they are made with a variety of fresh fruits. When you are unsure, ask about the ingredients used. Many juice bars use protein powder. Check to see if it is soy isolate, which has the highest concentrate of soy protein. If you are a regular customer, take your own soy protein powder and ask the server to add it to the smoothie.

Vegetarian Restaurants

There are now many vegetarian restaurants. While these restaurants offer meatless choices, the food is not always low-fat. Select menu items wisely, and inquire about cooking methods. Follow this same caution when selecting items marked "vegetarian" in regular restaurants. Be sure to ask what kinds of oils they are using. Avoid polyunsaturated fats.

Bagel Shops

Bagel shops are becoming popular in many areas of the country. Most have whole-grain bagels (avoid white flour bagels). Low-fat or nonfat spreads are usually available. Often cut-up fresh fruit or fruit juice is available.

Salad Bars

Choose generous amounts of a great variety of vegetables, fruit, and beans. For dressing, use vinegar and a small amount of olive oil. Choose saltine crackers to accompany your salad instead of croutons, which are often laden with fat. Say *no* to nuts and seeds, bacon bits, chopped egg, cheese. Avoid salads containing dressings, including mayonnaise. As a general rule, choose a broth-based vegetable soup over a cream soup, chowder, or a hearty meat soup.

Pizza Parlors

When ordering pizza in a traditional pizza parlor, ask for extra tomato sauce. Also ask for extra vegetables (onions, peppers, tomatoes, mushrooms) and no cheese. Choose whole-wheat crust when it is available. Upscale pizza parlors often have a variety of roasted vegetables available. Again, ask for extra tomato sauce and an abundance of vegetables. Say *no* to the sausage, pepperoni, cheese, olives, and anchovies.

Fast-Food Restaurants

It is difficult to follow the recommendations for prostate cancer when eating at fast-food restaurants and places that use prepared food items. If you can't avoid eating at these restaurants, do your homework. They all have nutrition information available for the asking. Learn which items at each of the restaurants best meet your needs. For instance, grilled chicken sandwiches (skip the mayonnaise or special sauce), salads (avoid the dressing or use fat-free dressing if it is available), or bean burritos make the best choices.

General Guidelines for Eating Out

Eating out was once described as the theater of the 1990s. It still is in the new millennium: your grand entrance as you sweep through the foyer; the scornful look of the maître d'; your waiter gleefully announcing himself with a broadcaster's

voice; the panache with which your wine arrives and is
corked. Sooooo, make your dietary needs known with a fla
Send a message to the chef via the wait staff that you want yo
meal to be as free of fat as possible. The bottom line for busin
is more people, more profit. If restaurants know that custom
want certain foods, they will prepare them or will stock the

For instance, say, "I have dietary concerns and need
food cooked without fat. I would like a grilled tomato wi
out Parmesan cheese," or "I need to have lots of vegetabl
Please give me a double portion of broccoli," or "I am try
to include more soy products in my menu plans. Please sto
canned soybeans and fresh green soybeans."

When you eat out or have someone else prepare yo
meals, you have less control over the outcome than when y
carefully select the freshest ingredients and fix the me
yourself. The guidelines that follow will help you stick
closely to the prostate cancer guidelines as possible. Here
some great ideas for you to select which should be availa
in most restaurants.

Breakfast Items

Fresh fruit	Oatmeal
Breadsticks	Grilled tomatoes
Fruit smoothie	Vegetable smoothie
Whole-grain cereal with nonfat milk or fruit juice	Fresh fruit

Soups

Tomato soup	Consommé
Broth-based vegetable soup	

Salads

Vegetable salads

Barley or bulgur salads
such as Tabouli

Bean or lentil salads

Fruit salads

Entrees

Pasta with tomato sauce

Vegetable whole-wheat
pizzas

Barley or bulgur dishes

Grilled, baked, broiled, or
poached fish or chicken
breasts

Bean burritos

Baked beans

Bean, lentil, or rice dishes

Stir-fry vegetables with tofu

Side Dishes

Baked or broiled tomatoes

Brown rice

Couscous

Roasted or steamed
vegetables

Vegetarian refried beans

Quinoa

Whole-grain pilafs

Baked sweet potatoes

Desserts

Angel food cake

Baked apple or pear

Sorbets, sherbets

Fresh fruit cup

Eating on the Run: *Gourmet on the Go*

Eating on the run has become a way of life for millions of
American men, myself included. If it takes more than a minute

to check out of an airport cafeteria line, I feel I've had to w
through a four-course meal. Face it, we just don't believe
have the time to eat properly anymore, and that forces us
pick up stuff that's nearly poison. I'm just appalled at
choices offered on most airlines, in most airports, in the m
bars of most hotels, and in fast-food stores. Even the salads a
vegetarian dishes are usually dripping with some godaw
mystery oil. It's hard to know whether it's left over from
engines. But fast does not need to be unhealthy. Here's a m
ern road warrior's guerrilla warfare guide to eating on the r

This is for the person who is too busy to cook and does
eat every meal at a restaurant. Make use of the now-availal
abundant selection of ready-to-use fresh vegetables, prepa
food items, and other quick-to-prepare foods. You may f
many of the foods recommended in this book in health fo
stores, such as Whole Foods, Fresh Fields, and Wild O.
However, they are available not only at specialty stores,
also in the produce section and at the deli counter in many
permarkets. These are rapidly expanding sections in the
permarket — make use of them and enjoy the variety offer

A little thought and planning will help you establish
inventory of foods to have on hand. On a trip to the su
market every week or two, you can stock up on food ite
you will need to put together meals with a minimum of t
and effort. Below is a shopping list that you can take w
you to the store. Buy some plastic containers and prep
your own MREs for the road. (*MRE* is the military term
meals ready to eat.) When you've traded in your frequ
traveler miles for a first-class seat, there's no greater joy t
turning away the "luxury" meal prepared by the airline
your own supermeal! You'll feel better than you ever belie
you could when you land. Compare that with the usual s

picious feeling that they just may be slowly poisoning you so you can't redeem any more miles! If you're going to take food with you on planes, make sure it's not perishable — you don't want to put yourself at risk for food poisoning.

SHOPPING LIST

Fresh washed and cut salad greens
Broccoli cole slaw
Other prepared vegetables
Cut-up fresh fruit and whole pieces of fresh fruit
Instant oatmeal
Whole-grain cereal
Nonfat milk or nonfat soymilk
Canned chopped tomatoes
Canned soybeans, other beans, baked beans
Tomato juice
Meatless spaghetti sauce with vegetables
Spaghetti noodles, whole wheat
Tomato puree
Tomato sauce
Baked tofu for sandwiches
Whole wheat bread or pita pockets
Packaged soups

Here are a few ideas to get you started:

- Sprinkle some dried cranberries, cherries, or raisins and a little wheat germ on prepared instant oatmeal.
- Have fruit spreads on bagels or whole-wheat toast.
- Use prepared salad greens, broccoli cole slaw mix, baby carrots, stir-fry mixes, and other prepared vegetables to make salad preparation quick and easy. Add canned beans

to salads. Try some of the flavored vinegars now on the market. Flavored vinegar with a little olive oil can liven up a bowl of greens and other vegetables. Keep a selection of flavored vinegars in your office (or your car if your car is your office!) so you can add them to vegetable salads.

- When putting together your evening meal, also package food for lunch the following day. When you are fixing vegetables for meals or on weekends, cook extra and take them with you for salads.

- Check out the variety of freeze-dried, instant soups available in cartons. Just add boiling water directly to the mix in the carton and wait a few minutes. Commonly available varieties include lentil, vegetable with pasta, bean, and split pea. These soups can be found in the gourmet section in supermarkets and at backpacking or outdoor recreational supply stores. (Beware of ramen-type noodle soups; they are often high in fat.) One easy way to meet the lycopene recommendation is to use these freeze-dried mixes as a foundation; add canned chopped tomatoes or substitute tomato puree for some of the boiling water.

- Make a quick sandwich with slices of baked tofu, lettuce, and tomato slices on whole-grain bread or into pita pockets. Or make a mixture of chopped lettuce and tomato with some beans to stuff into a pita pocket. Add some salsa and cilantro.

- Open a can of baked beans. Drain a can of soybeans and mix it with the baked beans, along with some tomato puree. Heat some of the mixture for dinner. Save some for dinner tomorrow or bring to work to heat up in the microwave.

- Heat up some spaghetti sauce from a jar while you boil

Dr. Bob's Handy Snack Ideas Requiring Little Preparation

Name	Sample Brand	Fat	Fiber	Sugar	Advantages
Three-grain bread	Mestemacher	2	6	0	Small cellophane wrapper, easy to take on trips.
Breakfast patties	The original Boca Breakfast patty	3	2	1	Great-tasting, just like real sausage, one minute in microwave.
Roasted vegetables in a pocket sandwich	Amy's	8	4	5	Quick microwave meal. I'll sometimes toss the crust.
Baby carrots	Bunny Love, organic peeled baby carrots				Come in an ideal small travel bag.
Vegetable blend	Cascadian Farm blend	0	0	4	Easy to microwave bag of great-tasting organic veggies, including broccoli, cauliflower, zucchini.
Wildberry muesli	Lifestream	3	5	10	Small box, easy to put in a briefcase.
Multigrain oat bran flakes	Nature's Path	<1	3	4	Sturdy transportable box.
Kashi, whole grains and sesame	Kashi Company	1	8	6	Super-healthy executive trail mix.
Organic brown rice miso	Miso Master				Neat plastic container, easy to transport.

Name	Sample Brand	Fat	Fiber	Sugar	Advantages
Teething biscuits	Healthy Times				Meant for teethers but oat and soy flour make it a great on-the-road snack.
Whole wheat pretzels	Harry's Whole Wheat Honeys	1.5	1	4	If you have to have pretzels, look for as much whole wheat as you can get. Whole wheat is is not the first ingredient, but they taste great.
Buckwheat noodles and miso broth	Westbrae Natural	0.5	2	1	Steamed, not fried! Fits in your briefcase and easy to cook with hotel-room hot water heater!
Whole wheat stone-ground sesame crackers	Ak-mak	2.2	3.5	2.3	Neat little package, super transportable.
Whole wheat couscous	Fantastic	1	7	0	Cooks in minutes and look at that fiber!
Black bean salsa couscous	Fantastic	1.5	8	6	These are nifty coffee-container-sized cups. Just add water and you're in business.
Veggie juice	Fresh Samantha				Pure carrot juice. National brand and widely available. Airplane-proof plastic container.
Cherry tomatoes					Portable and great tasting.
Cantaloupe sections					Portable way to take along fruit.
Dried fruits					Easiest way to carry fruit.
Other fresh fruits					

spaghetti noodles (whole wheat if possible). Put it all together and top with chopped fresh parsley.

- Pop a sweet potato or yam into a toaster oven or microwave to have for dinner.
- Serve whole wheat breadsticks to add crunch to a meal.
- Wash some grapes and put them on a cookie sheet in the freezer. When they are frozen, transfer to a plastic bag to store. They make great snacks.
- For dessert, have slices of angel food cake with fruit or sorbet.

Special Note for Women

There are very minor differences between the "his" and "her" diets for prostate and breast cancer prevention. You can prepare a variety of meals that will work perfectly for both of you. Here are the few minor differences:

- Experts are divided on the risks and benefits of fish oils for men. If male family members are at high risk, you may choose to limit the amount of fatty fish you serve.
- Some urologists restrict calcium intake in men already diagnosed with prostate cancer, whereas women need the calcium to maintain strong bones. For this reason, you may want to prepare foods low in calcium, but be certain that you and your daughters get the calcium you need by adding to your diet low-fat dairy products, calcium supplements, yogurt, and other high-calcium sources.
- The hallmark of the man's prostate-healthy diet is one very low in fat. In women, there is no indication, yet, that quantity of fat plays a role in breast cancer development. If males in your household are at high risk, you may want to consider the Asian and New American meal plans.
- The fat that is safest for both of you is olive oil.

Dr. Bob's Personal Strategy

Remember the slogan from our misspent youths, Better living through chemistry? Well, sometimes eating is so rushed, there's little more you can do than just pull the ingredients off the shelf and shove them down on the way out the door, much as you'd pour chemicals into a container. Occasionally, I scramble out of the house so fast in the morning for a *Today Show* appearance that I have time for 30 seconds of breakfast preparation and that's it. Here's what I do. Start your timers! Open the refrigerator door, pull out the low-fat yogurt, rip off the top of the container, pull the steel-cut oatmeal down from the cupboard, throw a little of each into a paper bowl, add raisins, raspberries, or blueberries, grab a plastic spoon, and head out the door. You can eat once you arrive at work, or if you're not driving, you can eat on the way. It's a super-nutritious breakfast that will hold you through the morning.

I'm not much of a chef and don't really care a great deal if I go out to a great restaurant. I see food as fuel, pure and simple — fuel that can dramatically improve my performance. I take a field-rations approach to eating — just get exactly what you need. I spend a lot of time each year on the road, including at least a month or two in places like Somalia, Kosovo, and Sudan. I just want what is necessary to keep performing my best. If you're like me and want a real no-nonsense approach, here it is. It's not perfect, but it gives you the basics.

PREWORKOUT MORNING SHAKE

40 grams soy

banana

ice

water

Optifuel II (a supplement made by Twinlab)

or

Fresh fruit

POSTWORKOUT BREAKFAST

Half cantaloupe

Whole-grain cereal with soymilk

Raspberries

Blueberries

LUNCH

Black bean soup

Swordfish steak

Four servings of fresh vegetables

V-8 juice

AFTERNOON SNACK

Sweet potato

DINNER

Black bean soup

Boca Burger

V-8 juice

Fresh veggies

See pages 253 to 269 for personal regimens of other men. You'll find programs and tips from Dr. Charles Myers, Mike Milken, and patients with prostate cancer.

Stress

After the publication of *The Breast Cancer Prevention Diet,* the question I heard the most often from women who had cancer was, "Why didn't you mention stress in your book?" They felt that more than any other factor, stress was responsible for their cancer. Many men, too, with prostate cancer mention harried and stressful business and personal lives as a potential causative factor, all in an age when everything seems to be moving too far too fast. I tell men and women who ask me about the stress-cancer connection that it's still way too early in the research to state emphatically that stress causes cancer. However, a recent report from the Far East may indicate that stress increases DNA oxidation, which is part of a process that can lead to genetic mutation. And a recent study from the State University of New York at Stony Brook indicated that men who had high amounts of stress in their lives were three times more likely to have high levels of an important prostate cancer marker than men with low stress; and men who lacked good supportive relationships with friends and family were twice as likely to have high levels of this same cancer marker as men with good social support. The most interesting observation is that those men with prostate cancer who engage in a program of stress reduction linked with regular exercise and a strict diet have the greatest success at lowering levels of this important prostate cancer marker. Without stress reduction, the program is far less effective. What is known is that stress does adversely affect the immune system, and it is the immune system that is one of the key defenses our body has against cancer. For that reason I've incorporated a major stress reduction program into my own life and into this book.

I visited with a group of men with prostate cancer who were participating in Dr. Ornish's study and asked them how anxious they were. These men were in a watchful-waiting program — their cancers had *not* been removed. Frankly, I expected them to be fearful. The group leader had one of those kind and gentle smiles that instantly put you at ease. She asked each of us in the group to say how we felt. When it was my turn, as a visitor, I said I felt both excited by what they were doing and somewhat on edge. To my great surprise, as the other men answered, the words they used were *satisfied, contented, grateful.* Huh? I was stunned, literally bowled over in my seat to hear in clear, calm tones just how incredibly relaxed and free of anxiety they were. I would have expected them to say: "I wake up at three in the morning in a cold sweat" or "I feel like I'm walking around under a cloud of doom during the day." Yet that was the exact opposite of what I heard. These men were about as centered as any group of men I had ever met. Each had an intimate sense of connection with those around the table. They each had a sense of peace so rarely seen in our crazed world — and they had achieved this peace through the foods they ate, through their regular group therapy, and through a powerful program of personal meditation that allowed them to slice their stress to a level more typical of a monk's. After meeting with these men who faced the real possibility of death and seeing the calm they showed, I understood that facing reality is not the problem — it's how you deal with it.

To see how stress can affect your immune defenses against cancer, let's take a brief look at the immune system.

Stress and the Immune System

The mind-body connection has always sounded like a lot of mumbo jumbo to me as it may have to many men. But when you look at the hard science, it's stunning to see how strong the connection is between the mind and the immune system. Consider this. White blood cells are a big part of the body's anticancer defense system. They have highly specialized names, such as T-lymphocytes, B-lymphocytes, macrophages, and natural killer cells. They are programmed to look for specific viruses, bacteria, and cancer cells. Although they very much have a mind of their own, like lonely sentries guarding a remote border they also have a high command-and-control that comes all the way down from the central nervous system. As in any bureaucracy, the commands are pretty general. Unfortunately, one of the central nervous system key commands can be to suppress the defense cells, making them far less effective, like a stand-down command from general headquarters. The command system the central nervous system uses is the body's hormones. Since this system goes from the brain through the central nervous system to the hormonal system to the immune system, the field of study is called psychoneuroimmunology.

The body's key stress hormone is cortisol. Cortisol is called a "stress hormone" because it coordinates the body's response to stress and orchestrates many other hormones and systems. How does cortisol work? White blood cells have receptors on them. As with other receptors mentioned in this book, think of those receptors as switches that are turned on by having a unique "key" placed in a matching lock. In this case the key is the stress hormone cortisol, and the lock is the receptor on the white blood cell; when the two connect, the immune system is turned down, like the dimmer switch for a light. This process is called down-regulation. It's known that cortisol weakens white blood cell function. Cortisol, in fact, is considered an immunosuppressant and is given to people after a kidney transplant so that their immune system does not reject the organ. Cortisol also blunts the immune system in patients with asthma or arthritis. What command causes the central nervous system to blunt the immune system? Stress!

Several studies confirm that stress turns down, or down-regulates, the immune system. Ronald Glaser, Ph.D., professor of molecular virology, immunology, and medical genetics, and his wife, professor of psychiatry Janice Kiecolt-Glaser, Ph.D., both at Ohio State University Medical Center, are top experts in the field of stress and immunology. In one study, Dr. Kiecolt-Glaser found that lonelier medical students had lower natural killer (NK) cell activity than their less-lonely fellow students.[1] And being married didn't help the immune system if the marriage had a lot of discord. Dr. Kiecolt-Glaser and colleagues conducted studies showing that marital conflict down-regulates immune function. In one study Dr. Kiecolt-Glaser examined problem-solving behaviors and immune function for 24 hours in 90 newlywed couples. She found that the couples who showed more negative or hostile behaviors during 30 minutes of discussing marital problems had over the 24 hours a greater decrease in their immune system function as measured by a decrease in their natural killer cells' ability to destroy threatening target cells. Also, the discussion of marital problems led to greater increase in blood pressure, which remained elevated longer in more negative subjects. Subjects who exhibited positive or supportive problem-solving behaviors had neither a down-regulated immune system nor an increased blood pressure.[2] When Dr. Kiecolt-Glaser and her colleagues conducted a similar study on older adults (couples with a mean age of 67 years) who had been married on average 42 years, she found similar results: the greater the marital conflict, the more down-regulated the immune system.[3]

The broader question is: what are the health implications? Researchers are now examining stress-induced immune changes, and their studies show surprising results.

The most practical way of seeing how constant stress affects your immune system is to observe whether you catch colds more easily. Dr. Sheldon Cohen and his colleagues at Carnegie Mellon University in Pittsburgh, Pennsylvania, inoculated people with 5 different forms of cold virus and found that psychological stress was related to whether they got cold symptoms and to the severity of the cold: the greater the psychological stress, the more severe the cold symptoms.

Dr. Kiecolt-Glaser and her colleagues examined the effects of chronic stress on spousal caregivers of patients with Alzheimer's disease. For 13 months she followed 69 spousal caregivers who had already been caring for their Alzheimer's-stricken partner for an average of 5 years. She compared the caregivers to a well-matched control group and found the caregivers to be at significantly greater health risk. The caregivers reported more days of infectious illness, especially upper respiratory tract infections. Caregivers also had a much greater occurrence of depressive disorders than controls. Caregivers with the least social support "showed the greatest and most uniform negative changes in immune function at follow-up."[4]

Now here's the interesting bottom line. Dr. Kiecolt-Glaser found that in spousal caregivers of patients with Alzheimer's, a wound took approximately 24 percent longer to heal than in well-matched controls.[5] The Glasers then conducted another study to examine the wound healing. They induced skin blisters by suction on the forearm of 36 women and found that women with higher stress had significantly lower levels of two key cytokines. Made by lymphocytes, cytokines are molecules that cells make to communicate with each other and promote healing. The two important cytokines that were found in much lower levels in stressed women were interleukin-1α and interleukin-8. In addition, those women with lower levels of cytokines had higher levels of cortisol in their saliva than women with higher cytokine levels.[6] This study suggested that psychological stress has a noticeable effect on cytokine production in the wound area.

Stress can even affect the immune system's response to vaccines. In one study looking at medical students' response to a vaccine, Dr. Glaser and Dr. Kiecolt-Glaser showed that academic stress could down-regulate the cellular immune response and affect the way the students responded to a viral vaccine. The Glasers and their colleagues found that stress inhibited both the antibody and virus-specific T cell (T-lymphocytes are a certain kind of white cell) responses to that vaccine; to get protection from the vaccine, you need both antibody and T cell response.[7] And in another study that looked at how stress affects immune response to immunization in older adults, the Glasers found that chronic stress altered the immune response to the influenza virus vaccine — both the antibody response and the virus-specific T-lymphocyte response were inhibited.[8]

Phew! All that said, more-frequent colds are a long way from cancer. Could stress actually be linked to cancer?

The Glasers have shown in a number of studies that psychological stress, distress, and depression can hinder repair of damaged DNA and alter apoptosis, or natural cell death. And since both repair of damaged DNA and apoptosis are important to cell health, inhibiting them could increase the risk of cancer.[9]

Harold G. Koenig, M.D., associate professor of psychiatry and medicine at Duke University, says: "Stress increases cortisol, and cortisol may influence interleukin-6 levels in the blood. High levels of interleukin-6 are indicative of an unstable immune system." These immune changes may increase susceptibility to certain forms of cancer.

Studies on stress and hormone-related tumors such as prostate cancer have not been done yet. Dr. Glaser hypothesizes: "If you have a hormone-related tumor (such as prostate cancer) and stress is modulating the hormones in such a way that the person is put at risk for developing the tumor, then, yes, we might be able to say that stress is affecting cancer. But these studies still need to be done."

So studies have still not conclusively demonstrated the link between stress and cancer. This does not mean, however, that you should not lower your stress levels in order to improve general health and potentially help prevent cancer. It's also unlikely that stress is the *only* factor in causing cancer.

What Is Stress?

Now let's take a closer look at what stress is and how to cut it.

"Stress evokes fight or flight," says Harvard University's Herbert Benson, M.D., father of the relaxation response. And the stress response appears whenever you're experiencing some type of danger to either your physical or your psychological self.

Dr. Glaser and Dr. Kiecolt-Glaser talk about defined

stressors; for example, academic stress or work stress or marital stress. "A stressor," says Dr. Glaser, "is something that would trigger in a person a physiological response that results in the activation of the hypothalamic-pituitary-adrenal (HPA) and sympathetic-adrenal-medullary (SAM) axes. HPA and SAM are two networks consisting of different organs that communicate through hormones such as cortisol or adrenaline or noradrenaline or growth hormones." So whatever is strong enough to activate HPA and SAM is a stressor.

All behavioral changes are stressful. There are two types of stressors: acute and chronic. An acute stressor is immediate, whereas a chronic one is long-term. We human beings are resilient animals and can withstand the acute stressors of everyday — for example, being stuck in traffic and arriving late to a meeting. Says Dr. Glaser: "These transitory acute stressors probably don't affect health risk. Hormonal changes do happen, and a few hours later hormone levels go back to normal; however, if those stressors continue over a long time, that has more implications for health. Also, genetic background, age, and gender will interplay more or less with those stressors to affect the immune system."

The opposite of the stress, or fight-or-flight, response is the relaxation response. Relaxation is a physiological state characterized by decreased metabolism, decreased heart rate, decreased blood pressure, decreased rate of breathing, and slower brain waves. Relaxation removes negative effects of stress, and the relaxation response is what you should be aiming for in your stress management program. Later in this chapter you'll find a discussion of techniques that evoke the relaxation response — for example, meditation, prayer, yoga, tai chi, and qigong. You may have heard the phrase "relaxation response" before and it does have a tired ring to it, *but* once you've truly experienced it, you'll be amazed. The true relaxation response brings you back down to ground zero in terms of stress. Seriously, you'll find yourself more calm than you ever believed you could be, even when at the heart of a major crisis.

Cutting Stress

To manage stress effectively in your life, you'll probably need to include several elements in your plan. Of course, you should individualize your program for your particular need, but make sure you incorporate at least the essential blocks listed below. If you're having trouble establishing and maintaining a stress management program, consult your physician and try to make stress management part of an ongoing relationship with your doctor, from whom you can also get support and guidance. The best high concept to remember about stress is this: "Stress is a habit. Responding in a stressful way is a habit that is learned and you can unlearn it, but it requires repetition and success and reinforcement," according to David Larson, M.D., president of the National Institute for Healthcare Research and adjunct professor in the Department of Psychiatry at Duke Medical Center and Northwestern Medical School.

Here are the key components of the program. Remember, those techniques that really bring the stress levels down are the ones that engage the mind-body connection most fully. That's why you will find longer sections on meditation and prayer.

Mind-Body Programs

Prostate cancer patients in Dean Ornish's nutrition trial practice yoga and meditation as part of the study. I met them at a church high above Sausalito, California, in the scene described in the introduction to this chapter. Says Dr. Ornish: "We ask them to spend a total of one hour per day doing meditation, yoga, and other stress management techniques. We teach them to meditate in a way that's comfortable with their own religious or secular beliefs. It's not all or nothing; the more you do the more benefits you receive." That may seem like an extravagant amount of time. But if there is one lesson I've learned from Dr. Ornish over the years, it is this: you can try to "manage" stress or you can simply reset your stress levels to zero. "When people meditate and practice yoga, they often say that their fuse gets longer," says Dr. Ornish. "Things just don't bother them as much." I long thought that was impossible but was finally able to achieve it through a prolonged session of yoga called Bikram's yoga. True, you can't keep stress at zero unless you live in a monastery, but what you can do is recall the feeling of peace and hold on to the sense of calm throughout your stressful day.

Bikram's Yoga

Okay! If you're like me, you may not be able to sit still long enough to meditate. I'll admit I never could — until I found a relatively new kind of yoga called Bikram's yoga. I do it. You'll find it quite strenuous, but Bikram's yoga will wipe your emotional slate cleaner than will any other method I've tried to date. If you're doubtful, just try a single class and see if your stress hasn't been erased. The Web site www.bikramyoga.com has all the information you'll need. What I love best is the way you lean into a muscle. The stretch is incredible, highly aerobic, causing long, wonderful, deep breaths. Each time you think you've hit a hard end to your stretch, the muscle gives a little more. Yoga literally changes your body and the way you feel about yourself. It's also a great way to rehabilitate an aging body, giving it new flexibility and freedom from the aches and pains that come with the forties, fifties, and beyond. Rather than concentrating on a word, you concentrate on each breath. The idea is actually quite exotic, that you are inhaling energy from the universe. If you've had trouble meditating, you'll find that concentrating on the intense physical experience and the wonderful long, deep breaths is amazing.

Once you've experienced the deep sense of relaxation, you can call on it at times of stress. I'll find my shoulders and neck tightening when I'm stressed. I'll take a deep breath and summon up a relaxation response and presto, the tension is gone! Honest! I can't emphasize strongly enough how powerful a technique this is, truly one that can transform your life. And if you say you're too inflexible, well, the more inflexible the better. Why? You have that much more for your muscles to pull against. That means you'll get much more out of a workout, and over the long term you'll make much more progress!

Traditional Meditation

The relaxation response can also be achieved through meditation that draws on many techniques within the old Eastern and Western religious traditions of Christianity, Judaism, Buddhism, and Hinduism. Physicians throughout the country are now using meditation and other relaxation response techniques in their treatment of patients. Christina Puchalski, M.D., assistant professor of internal medicine at George Washington University and director of education at the National Institute for Healthcare Research, offers the following guidelines for meditation.

First, select a word that is spiritual to you (e.g., peace, love, light, one). If you're religious, choose a word from your religious tradition; for example, "Christ" or "ohm" ("ohm" comes from the Hindu tradition). In Christianity this practice is called "the centering prayer." Father Thomas Keating, Cistercian monk and a priest at St. Benedict's Monastery in Snowmass, Colorado, was one of the founders of both the centering prayer movement, which started around 1975, and Contemplative Outreach, which is an organization designed to support those introduced to centering prayer. Centering prayer is largely based on *The Cloud of Unknowing*, written by an unknown English fourteenth-century spiritual guide who, in teaching a contemplative kind of prayer to a disciple, said: "Choose a word, a simple word, a single-syllable word is best, like *God* or *love*, but choose a word that is meaningful to you."

Now find a quiet place for yourself. Choose a comfortable chair and sit with good posture, back erect, feet uncrossed and firmly on the ground, and eyes closed. If you feel more comfortable on a cushion, sit cross-legged on a cushion, but make sure you keep your back straight.

Breathe slowly and deeply, in and out, in and out. While you're exhaling or breathing out, utter either silently or loudly the chosen word. Continue doing this for the amount of time that you're meditating. Focus all of your attention on the word. When thoughts cross your mind, don't engage them or hold on to them; just let them go by bringing your attention back to your word. (To become highly skilled at deep breathing, take a yoga class that concentrates on breathing — you'll be amazed just how well it works.)

At the end of your meditation time, slowly open your eyes.

When you first start to meditate, you'll notice that your

mind is busy, that thoughts keep popping up. Don't worry, let them go, focus again on the word, and you'll find that your mind will gradually quiet. Don't be impatient. It takes time and practice to learn to still your mind. At first, practice for 5 minutes a day. Do not set an alarm, but keep a clock nearby so that you can see it if you open your eyes after 1 minute. Start with 5 minutes and build up to what Dr. Benson recommends based on his studies — 10 to 20 minutes once or twice a day.

Studies show benefits of meditation and other relaxation response techniques for PMS, anxiety, depression, heart disease, high blood pressure, chronic pain, and headache.

Qigong

For physically active men, I also like qigong (pronounced chi gung). Like acupuncture, qigong is an actual Chinese medical art that has been around for thousands of years. Qigong involves wonderful slow, rhythmic physical movement coupled with deep breathing and meditation, really the best of all worlds. There is a growing body of scientific literature demonstrating its effectiveness, for instance in lowering blood pressure. A few paragraphs here really don't do justice to these techniques, which is why I advise you do what I did — take several classes to get started. I've found even a single class is enough to give you the basics and tell you whether this technique will work for you. More than anything, I think you'll be impressed with a real sense of inner peace, far more powerful than any drugs for anxiety. If you take a few classes, then try qigong at home but have trouble maintaining concentration, continue taking classes. Since you know you're stuck for the length of the class, you'll be much more likely to just let go and lose yourself in the class.

Prayer

Scientific studies now show that prayer works wonders on health. Of the 300 studies on spirituality in scientific journals, the National Institute of Health Research found 75 percent showed that religion and prayer have a positive effect on health. Practicing your religious or spiritual belief will be extremely beneficial to your health. In fact, religion is one of the most powerful health measures there is. Consider this:

A recent study by Dr. Robert A. Hummer at the University of Texas in Austin found that attending religious services more than once a week could increase your life expectancy by 7 years or, if you are African American, potentially 14 years![10] Another study, made by Dr. Harold G. Koenig and colleagues at Duke University's Center for the Study of Religion/Spirituality and Health, found that in 3,968 community-dwelling adults aged 64 to 101, frequent attenders of religious services had a 46 percent decreased risk of dying during the 6-year follow-up in comparison to infrequent attenders.[11] So one of the single most powerful health measures there is, is becoming religious. That's measured by this stunning increase in longevity.

A Dartmouth Medical School study found that of 232 patients who underwent elective heart surgery, the very religious were three times more likely to recover than those who were not. The most consistent indicator of survival was the amount of strength or comfort the patients said they received from their religious faith. In fact, the more religious they described themselves as being, the greater the protective effect. Of 37 patients who described themselves as "deeply religious," none died. The researchers also found that the more socially active patients had higher survival rates. More time spent in religious activity correlated with more overall happiness and satisfaction.[12]

Dr. Harold G. Koenig discovered that "the likelihood of having a diastolic blood pressure of 90 or higher, the level most often associated with increased risk for strokes or heart attacks, was 40 percent lower among those who attended a religious service at least once a week and prayed or studied the Bible at least once a day, than among those who did so less often."[13] In another study with the elderly, Dr. Koenig and David Larson, M.D., found that people 60 and older who attended religious services at least once a week were 56 percent less likely to have been hospitalized in the previous year than those attending services less frequently.[14] In fact, the health measure that leads to the greatest longevity *is* religion.

How does religion work? Partly it is obvious: many religions, such as the Church of Jesus Christ of Latter-day Saints, promote better health habits. Partly it is that religion delivers the power of being part of a community. But perhaps the most powerful factor is the sense of optimism that it gives you, according to research by Professor Martin Seligman at the University of Pennsylvania. He says:

> We found that the more authoritarian religions produce more hope and optimism. The questionnaire and analysis of sermons and liturgy showed that fundamentalist individuals were significantly more optimistic and hopeful than moderates, who in turn were more optimistic and hopeful than liberal individuals. The more frequently people participated in fundamentalist religious activities, the less likely they were to report emotional distress. A causal model that takes into account religious influence in daily

life and the effects of religious involvement, religious hope, and religious liturgy on explanatory style seems to account exhaustively for the effect of fundamentalism on optimism.

Of course the more religious people might have been more optimistic to start out, but religion only strengthened their optimism. And as we've seen, a positive explanatory style is incredibly potent, performing as well as drugs in the treatment of depression and obsessive-compulsive disorder.

Patients, say the experts, respond to prayer because it offers hope, a way to cope, a sense of peace, and an overall sense of well-being. Prayer also works as a form of meditation, counteracting stressful thoughts while lowering heart rate and breathing, slowing brain waves, and relaxing muscles. In one study, Dr. Harold Koenig measured interleukin-6 levels in a church group. High levels of interleukin-6 usually indicate an unstable immune system as we have seen, and the church group members had lower interleukin-6 levels, suggesting enhanced immune function. In fact, people who attended religious services were only half as likely to have high levels of interleukin-6 in their bloodstream as nonattenders.

"I don't think we should just be looking at prayer and religious commitment; we should also look at spirituality in the more general sense of the term," Dr. David Larson says. By spirituality, Dr. David Larson means a relationship to the transcendent that gives meaning and purpose to your life; this can be a divine being, God, or something else, such as nature, an energy force, or even art. "Spirituality seems to be helped by a structure," Dr. Larson says; in other words, if you are practicing your spirituality with others within a belief system (e.g., going to church or synagogue or mosque), you seem to be able to reap greater health benefits. "We should look first at spirituality, then at religious or spiritual commitment, and then at the role of prayer in spiritual or religious commitment."

Prayer is communication with the absolute, the divine, o God. This communication can take two forms: prayer a speaking to God or meditation as contemplating or listenin to God or the divine.

Develop Your Own Spiritual Program

Although the choice of a specific faith is not a medical but personal decision, several physicians now actually recommend that people incorporate spirituality in their lives. "I en courage a spiritual program consisting of a) prayer, b reading of scripture, c) worship attendance, and d) involve ment with a faith community," says Dale A. Matthew M.D., author of *The Faith Factor* and former professor medicine at Georgetown University School of Medicine.

Prayer: Although I can't create a formula for you because d tails of prayer are individually based, try to pray every da

Reading of scriptures: Whatever your faith, read some sacre scripture every day.

Worship attendance: If you have religious belief, attend a r ligious service at least once a week.

Involvement with a faith community: Become involved wi a worship community; find a comfortable place. People worship communities help and encourage one another throu good and bad times.

If you have this impulse, then practicing your religious spiritual belief will be extremely beneficial to your health.

you don't, try using meditation by itself. Of course the religious or spiritual impulse must first come out of deeply held beliefs that are beyond the scope of this book. If you are spiritual, you'll find that if you suffer the endless, nagging uncertainty of life in our modern age, you can be vastly reassured by trust in a higher being.

Many of us relate religion to fear, guilt, and dread. I had dinner with several Trappist monks, whom I expected to be unusually stern and severe. To the contrary, they were intoxicated with their sense of spiritual connection. They had achieved a state of spiritual awareness that evoked admiration and awe.

Visualization

Visualization is a great option for a mind-body program if you can't manage to or don't have the inclination to pray or meditate. Guided imagery asks you to visualize whole scenes. You can buy tapes that help you visualize. Martin Rossman, M.D., has an excellent series of tapes, as does Dr. Andrew Weil.

Other Stress Busters

While you'll want to consider some mind-body program to bring an overall sense of peace and tranquillity, these additional measures are powerful stress busters that you may want to add.

Nutrition

Foods are huge stressors. Many of us create our own chronic fatigue–like syndromes by eating refined foods that wreak havoc with our blood sugar levels and by drinking too much caffeine, which gives us surges of adrenaline and blood sugar throughout the day. We then use alcohol to become unstrung, sealing a vicious cycle. By following the meal plans in this book, you'll feel a great deal more calm. Consider eliminating caffeine, refined-flour carbohydrates, alcohol, and tobacco as well as cocaine, marijuana, and other recreational drugs if you use them. They may give you immediate symptomatic relief, but they crank up the physical and psychological stress on your system. If you find it difficult to give up junk foods, you'll find that cutting your stress through the measures in this chapter will go a long way toward cutting your craving for them! I swear I've gained another four hours a day of productivity just by avoiding foods that stress me out, especially starchy and refined carbohydrates.

Sleep

Sleep deprivation will most certainly make you feel more stressed. Although there is great variation in how much sleep men say they need, lesser amounts of sleep are associated with poorer health and poorer longevity. For great sleep preparation techniques, consult my book *The Biology of Success* or a specialist in sleep disorders.

Physical Activity

Exercise has the fastest and most dramatic effect on stress. Your exercise routine should include both an aerobic and a stretching/deep-breathing routine.

Aerobic Exercise: When we're stressed, our stress hormone levels and adrenaline hormone levels go up. Dr. Puchalski has shown that aerobic exercise lowers these stress hormone levels.

For aerobic exercise, you need to do vigorous exercise

that gets your heart rate up. Dr. Puchalski recommends that her patients exercise 30 minutes 3 times a week.

Stretching and Deep Breathing: Deep breathing has been shown to evoke what Dr. Benson calls the relaxation response, and that's why I've discussed yoga and qigong above in the section on the mind-body programs.

In a study, Bonnie G. Berger and David R. Owen compared mood benefits of different types of exercise and found that what is important may be the abdominal breathing and not the aerobic component of exercise. They reported that "stress-reduction benefits of hatha yoga were similar to those previously reported for jogging and swimming."[15]

Yoga, tai chi, and qigong all offer great deep breathing. You can also stretch and deep-breathe even while you're at your desk. Dr. Puchalski suggests to her patients that even while they're sitting at a desk, they should stop their work for a few minutes, take deep breaths, and rotate their shoulders and move their head from side to side. Count 4 to 5 repetitions.

Massage

To reap the benefit of massage, you should do it on a regular basis, depending on what you can afford — once a week or once a month. Make sure, however, that you go to a certified massage therapist (CMT) who knows what he or she is doing and won't injure you.

Herbal Teas

Herbal teas such as chamomile, passionflower, valerian, or American ginseng are great for relaxing.

Aromatherapy

Researchers are exploring and discovering the benefits of aromatherapy for, among other things, insomnia, anxiety, weight loss, pain management, concentration problems, and heart ailments.

RELAXING AROMAS

Lavender
Ylang ylang (ylang ylang is a tropical flower that grows in Malaysia and Indonesia)
Roses
Chamomile
Geranium
Sandalwood
Frankincense
Jasmine

My book *The Biology of Success* has a thorough guide on how to apply aromatherapy.

Music Therapy

Yes, sound heals. Music therapy is being used effectively for changing patients' moods. If you want to consult a music therapist, make sure he or she is board certified — the initials MT–BC will appear after the therapist's name. The American Music Therapy Association is based in Maryland.

There are lots of great CDs of music for relaxation. I especially like Don Campbell's *The Mozart Effect,* Volume 2, "Heal the Body: Music for Rest and Relaxation." For a comprehensive discussion of music therapy, see my book *The Biology of Success.*

Miscellaneous

- Find what works to relieve your stress; it can be baths or heating pads, or great sex.
- Petting animals. Studies show that if you pet animals, especially cats, your blood pressure goes down.

If you're constantly feeling stressed and depressed or anxious, you should consult your physician to discuss psychotherapy and/or medication options.

You'll find that pursuing the programs in this chapter may make the most dramatic difference of all in how you feel and perform in day-to-day life. How much do you need to do? In Dr. Ornish's program, men spend a full hour on relaxation techniques. You may say, "How in my crazy life can I ever find that kind of time?" I've found that investing that hour a day pays me back with hours more of concentrated mental energy. But as Dr. Ornish says, "When I get very busy, I play a little game with myself. I say, 'Do I have one minute to meditate?' I can usually find one minute — otherwise, I'd have to admit my life is way out of balance. If I do it for a minute, then I'll usually do it for longer; getting started is always the most difficult part. But even a minute a day has real benefits. The consistency is more important than the duration. More is better, but try to do a little every day."

Exercise

Ralph Paffenbarger is one of the most legendary epidemiologists of our time. He was the first to demonstrate conclusively many of the effects of exercise on longevity, risk of heart disease, and sudden death. Physicians have long relied on his studies as information you could bank on. It's no surprise that he was one of the first to develop data on prostate cancer and exercise.

Dr. Paffenbarger showed that men over 70 who consistently maintained high levels of exercise lowered their risk of prostate cancer by 50 percent. How much exercise? The study showed these benefits were seen among those who expended more than 4,000 calories a week versus those who expended less than 1,000 calories a week.[1] Furthermore, Edward Giovannucci, M.D., at Harvard, examined physical activity and prostate cancer in male health professionals registered in the Health Professionals Follow-Up Study and found that men who exercised at high levels — at least 3 hours of vigorous exercise per week — were only around half as likely to be diagnosed with metastatic prostate cancer.

What possible relationship could exercise have to prostate cancer? The most prevalent theory is that high levels of physical activity lower acutely and chronically the levels of testosterone circulating in the blood. Dr. A. C. Hackney and others showed that a long bout of exercise can cause a rise in testosterone during the workout, followed by a drop. If the activity was for more than two hours, the reduction in testosterone was anywhere from 25 to 50 percent! Men with endurance training had resting total testosterone levels that were only 60 to 85 percent of levels in untrained men of the same age.[2] Different studies — by T. Buss, K. Häkkinen, and G. D. Wheeler — all show that 1 to 6 months of exercise training produced a significant lowering of testosterone levels.[3] In Dr. Wheeler's study, men who adopted a 6-month exercise regimen that culminated in running an average of 35 miles a week had around a 30 percent reduction in total testosterone.

Why would lower testosterone levels potentially affect prostate cancer? Because prostate cancer is sensitive to testosterone and other male sex hormones (androgens), as we saw in the chapter on soy. When physicians withdraw androgen stimulation through hormone therapy, the prostate cancer often regresses. Castrates, who have abnormally low testosterone levels, almost never have prostate cancer.[4] P. H. Gann showed that testosterone levels, even in the low-normal range — in other words, at a level that physical exercise could affect — could lower the risk of prostate cancer.[5] My first reaction to this was, hey, great, but what about my sex life — wouldn't less testosterone affect my sex life? Researchers have reassured me that dropping from high to normal levels of testosterone has no effect on our virility.

Dr. P. H. Gann offers another hypothesis as to why exercise might affect prostate cancer risk. He suggests in a study that exercise reduces the release of growth factors that stimulate epithelial cell division in the prostate.[6]

While these studies show that physical activity reduces prostate cancer risk,[7] there are other studies that fail to find a relationship, perhaps because the exercise was of lower intensity or for a shorter duration of time.[8] Studies still need to determine the required type of workout, intensity, duration, and frequency of physical exercise, and whether there is a certain period in a man's life when exercising is particularly beneficial. Since physical activity, however, is such an easil alterable risk factor and since physical activity promotes general health, it's part of the Prostate Cancer Protection Pro gram.

Exercise has many general anticancer effects: it improv general immune function and antioxidant defenses, chang the time of digestion, regulates blood sugar, and lowers bod fat. We know for sure that increased antioxidant defense an lower fat intake are protective against prostate cancer. In a dition, exercise elevates mood and may therefore prote against disease through psychological well-being and efficie stress management.

Dr. Paffenbarger's general recommendation for over great health is, "People should expend 1,500 to 2,000 kil calories per week. They should have 2 moderately vigoro stints of activity each week." Dr. Paffenbarger adds that you're younger you should aim for a little more activity, a if you're older, a little less. I push myself hard. Consideri that preliminary studies indicate exercise at a high level beneficial, I aim for a minimum of 10 hours of vigorous a obic activity a week.

Your Guide to Physical Activity

Choosing an Exercise

I find the best exercises are the ones that you can do longest and hardest. Say you're aiming to burn 4,000 calo a week. Sure, if you're an Olympic oarsman you could kn it off in two and a half hours of high-intensity rowing 1,500 calories per hour. But at a slow walk, that could t you ten hours! Ouch! For that reason I like exercises that can offer a minimum load on the joints and ligaments yet a maximum impact on major muscle groups. Cycling is a perfect example. On a bike you can almost go forever. More practically, you can cruise along in a trance for hours at a time, yet you can also suddenly hammer at high intensity with little of the risk of injury found in high-impact sports such as aerobic dance. Recumbent stationary bikes have the lowest load of all! Stair machines, cross-country ski machines, spinning machines, and treadmills are the twenty-first-century tranquilizer. Nearly always available, they're a great stress breaker in the middle of the day and a great way to pick up energy in the mid- to late afternoon.

Intensity

I find vigorous exercise far more effective than moderate exercise for lowering my tension level and making me feel better for the rest of the day. Vigorous exercise is also the best way to control your weight because it puts your body into a fat-burning phase for several hours after the workout. Be sure to check with your doctor before you begin a vigorous training program.

How Much

Benefits just keep increasing as you increase the length and intensity of the workout. Some experts believe that in order to reap the full health benefits of exercise, you will need to exercise vigorously for four hours every week. Many men, like my editor, think that's a lot. But stop for a minute and think of Jack Lalanne's philosophy of two hours of hard exercise a day. He's now well into his eighties and is living proof of the concept.

Fitness Levels

Fitness is a continuous variable — we can talk about high, very high, extremely high fitness, et cetera, but you can make these distinctions between moderate and high fitness:

Moderate Fitness: If you run a few miles several times a week, you're moderately fit. Thirty minutes of brisk walking will also get you out of the low-fit and into the moderately fit category. Brisk walking means being able to walk one mile in 15 to 20 minutes. A well-balanced moderate fitness program would include, at minimum, a) 30 minutes of brisk walking every day — you can accumulate that in three 10-minute walks, and b) two or three times a week some weight lifting and stretching or other activities that condition the muscles.

High Fitness: To be highly fit, you have to exercise more than 30 minutes a day every day — this could mean running/jogging for 30 or more minutes, or doing moderate-level exercise for more than 30 minutes every day. Dr. Steven Blair of the Cooper Institute says that running anywhere from 20 to 50 miles a week would put you in the highly fit category. Even at 40 to 50 miles a week, there is no increased risk of premature mortality, although people who run that much are more likely to experience bone and joint injuries and may also be more likely to impair their immune function. If you'd rather bike, blade, cross-country ski, swim, hike, or power walk, then for high fitness you would need up to an hour of vigorous exercise per day.

If you're going for more than moderate fitness, be sure to get a good evaluation and recommendations from an orthopedic surgeon who practices sports medicine to be sure you aren't going to damage ligaments, joints, or tendons by going too hard or too fast. And if you have risk factors for heart disease or are over fifty, be sure to consult a cardiologist before undertaking any rigorous exercise programs.

Exercise Environment

Always wondered why it's harder to exercise indoors? Jane Harte and George Eifert found in a study that the group that exercised outdoors had the most positive moods during and following exercise, while those who exercised indoors and had no external stimuli showed the least positive affect, and, in fact, showed a negative mood following the exercise bout.[9] Environment also affects the runner's biology: indoor and outdoor runners showed different patterns of urinary adrenaline, noradrenaline, and cortisol excretion. In their study on swimming and yoga, Bonnie Berger and David Owen also found that an uncomfortable exercise surrounding can actually have a negative effect on mood; when swimmers exercised in a too-warm water temperature of 106°F, their mood became negative. If you have to exercise indoors, as many of us do, you can still boost your mood by exercising with a class, boosting your spirits with music, or finding a gym with lots of windows facing onto the great outdoors.

Mood

Finally, the hormones adrenaline, noradrenaline, and cortisol all rise with regular exercise. During depression, levels decrease, which led researchers to conclude that these hormones are instrumental in the positive effect of exercise on mood. Exercise also increases brain blood flow, thus allowing more oxygen into the brain, which is key to improving mental energy, especially after waking in the morning or after an afternoon nap.

WHAT YOU CAN DO NOW

First meet with your doctor to check your heart health
general health, and then lay out an exercise plan and stic
it. Aim for 3 hours of vigorous aerobic exercise a week.
activities count — tennis, Rollerblading, and mountain
ing are all great ways to keep fit.

You should refrain from exercise, particularly cyc
(since it stimulates the prostate), for at least 3 days before
ting a prostate checkup because exercise might artific
increase your PSA, the prostate cancer marker discusse
Part IV.

Part Four

Protection

The main thrust of this book is that nutrition and lifestyle changes are the best, safest, and most accessible means of protecting yourself against prostate cancer . . . but that's not all! Let's look at the other key ways of protecting yourself.

• First, screening. A simple blood test can warn you of a problem long before it becomes serious, if you begin testing when you are young enough. That test is called the PSA test.

• Second, PSA tracking. By plotting your PSA on a regular basis, you can detect the earliest possible hint of trouble. Major research groups are also using PSA tracking as a way of following the effectiveness of foods, diets, and supplements.

• Third, chemoprotection. There is a major push to find a prostate cancer prevention pill. Since public health officials realize that many Americans will never change their diet, they are looking for a once-a-day medication that could prevent the disease. We'll look at several examples that are now in the pipeline.

• Fourth, surgery. Surgeons are constantly innovating and looking for new surgical approaches with fewer side effects. Here we'll take a look at how to get the best possible results.

Early Warning: The PSA Test

Remember as kids in school hearing about the DEW line? It was a highly sophisticated radar system strung across the Arctic to warn the American military that the Soviet Union was sending airplanes or missiles to attack the United States. As technology grew, satellite surveillance of missile silos in Russia increased our ability to detect an imminent attack even earlier. Now the Pentagon can even track the transfer of plutonium into rogue countries where terrorists might use the plutonium to make a bomb. Military analysts want the earliest warning they can get. They know the earlier the warning, the better they can protect America. The same is true in prostate cancer. Early detection can protect you from having a cancer ever get to the size where it could hurt you. The early-warning test for prostate cancer is a blood test called the PSA test, and it *can* warn you *before* you actually get into trouble — if you take it early enough. Detecting even a hint of trouble early on allows you to take charge, using the protective measures you've read about in this book. That's the big picture, and that's why PSA is an important part of this book. In this chapter we'll look at the test itself, when to take it, and how to use it. In the next chapter we'll look at a new use of the test called "tracking PSA." It may be the best early-warning system of all and is the ideal way to use PSA along with this book.

What Is the PSA Test?

Prostate Specific Antigen (PSA) is a perfectly normal and healthy body protein produced by the prostate. PSA's role has always been a bit of a mystery. The best guess is that it breaks down coagulated semen. New research shows it may also have some natural cancer-fighting activity. While normal prostate cells produce PSA, so do cancerous ones. The difference is that cancer can produce tremendous amounts of PSA, whereas the normal prostate does not. That means that PSA could serve as a signal that you have prostate cancer. Of course there is no practical way of reaching into the prostate and measuring how much PSA is there. Fortunately, PSA leaks into the bloodstream. Its appearance in the blood gives us a unique window into what's happening within the prostate. Usually only a small amount of PSA leaks into the blood, but when for some reason the prostate gears up its production of PSA, lots more appears in the blood as well, making PSA a pretty good barometer of trouble. I say pretty good because cancer is not the only cause of a rising PSA. For instance, a needle biopsy or ejaculation can temporarily increase PSA levels in the blood. Also, age and a condition called benign prostatic hypertrophy increase the amount of prostate tissue, which causes PSA levels to rise. Prostate cancer, however, causes the most dramatic increase in PSA.

The PSA test measures PSA in the bloodstream, and the measurement is nanograms per milliliter of serum (ng/ml). A nanogram is one billionth of a gram, a pretty minute amount. The PSA test is usually done along with a digital rectal exam (DRE), a test during which your urologist will insert his finger into your rectum to feel for abnormalities in the prostate. The digital rectal exam is conducted along with the PSA test because the combination of the two tests provides a more accurate diagnosis than either test alone. How good is it? PSA alone is the most powerful test in cancer today. The combination of the PSA and DRE tests is a much more powerful predictor of cancer than the mammogram is in breast cancer, and that says quite a lot. If both PSA and DRE are positive, there is a very high likelihood that you do have cancer.

When to Start Testing

There are more and more anecdotal reports of men who have a PSA performed as part of a routine physical exam only to learn, to their shock and dismay, that they have advanced prostate cancer. "If only I had been tested earlier," they say. Peter Albertsen, M.D., of the University of Connecticut Health Center in Farmington, reports that some are suing doctors. Why? They're claiming that if they had been screened earlier they could have been saved! Don't be one of them! Below are current guidelines by specialists for when to start testing. The age at which you first begin testing is determined by whether you are at high or low risk. If you don't know your risk, please refer to Appendix One: How to Determine Your Risk of Prostate Cancer (page 273).

Keep in mind that the public health community does *not* advocate early testing, because of the huge cost to the health care system. However, the test is cheap, about $15. If you're willing to pay for it yourself, most urologists see no objection. I like early testing because it gets you in at the ground floor. That is, you are highly likely to find a PSA that is within the normal range. If you see your PSA begin to rise or climb near the danger zone in subsequent tests, you have many more options open to you to protect yourself. You'll hear lots of controversy about the PSA test. There's a full discussion in the appendix. But most of that controversy has to do with cost. It you're footing the bill, the choice is yours. Opponents also say that there's not enough evidence to prove that men's lives are being saved since the test hasn't been around long enough to prove that point. But as we'll see, cancers are being found at a much earlier stage than would have been possible before the test became available.

Age 35 with Very High Risk

Get your first PSA test at age 35 if you have a *very* strong family history of prostate cancer. "Men with a family history or African-American men should have their first test at age 35," recommends E. David Crawford, M.D., professor of urology and radiation oncology at the University of Colorado. Appendix One details which men are at higher risk and why. Fortunately, an extremely small number of men will have cancer at this age. Robert Krane, M.D., director of neurology at Massachusetts General Hospital, says: "I've only seen one man in his 30s — and he was 39 — with prostate cancer." Just as women with a high risk for breast cancer get their first base-line mammogram test at age 35, men at very high risk for prostate cancer should consider 35 a baseline from which to gauge the results of further testing.

Age 40 with High Risk

This is the age at which most experts recommend a first test for men at high risk. You could consider a baseline test as part of a personal protection strategy, since the chances are excellent that your result would be well within the normal limit.

Age 45: Baseline

Dr. Crawford recommends age 45 for a first screening for men not at high risk. At this age, it's likely that most men who are not at high risk will still have a PSA that is well within the normal range. This is the age when most men can get a decent baseline.

Age 50: Recommended Age for Regular Testing

PSA advocates recommend that all men over 50 get tested. This is the conventional age for most men to have their first test and to begin annual screening.

What Your Score Means

PSA Greater Than 10

If you have a PSA of over 10, the likelihood of cancer is extremely high. Researchers estimate that 70 to 80 percent of men with abnormal digital rectal exams and PSA levels over 10 have prostate cancer. Your doctor will probably follow up with ultrasound and biopsy to determine if you have cancer.

PSA 4 to 10

If you have a PSA between 4 and 10 and a normal rectal exam, you have a 25 to 30 percent chance of having cancer. This is the "gray" area in prostate cancer testing. Doctors expend a lot of effort trying to discern among those in the 4 to 10 range who has cancer and who doesn't. If your PSA is over 4 and you have a palpable mass on your rectal exam or a PSA that is going up, your doctor will recommend a biopsy. The urologist inserts a half dozen or so small needles into the prostate and removes small pieces of tissue. Those are examined under the microscope for signs of cancer. An alternative is to be followed more closely with frequent PSAs and for the doctor to examine your prostate with a very high quality new color ultrasound for evidence of cancer. The good news is that just having an elevated PSA doesn't mean you have prostate cancer. There are other explanations, such as age, benign prostatic hypertrophy, or even infection. A number of corroborative tests have been developed to improve the diagnostic accuracy of the PSA test, lower your anxiety, and reduce the expense of unnecessary biopsies. These tests could save you from having a biopsy. There's a full description of them in Appendix Three.

PSA 2 to 4

Two to 4 has long been considered within the normal range for PSA, but that does not mean your PSA will stay normal for long. If you have the recommended yearly testing, look what happens to PSA. At the end of three years, 35 percent of men with PSAs between 2 and 4 had a PSA that had risen higher than 4, Dr. Crawford found in a study of 8,000 men. So if you're in the 2 to 4 range, you still need to be followed closely. Some doctors think that 4 is too high a cutoff. Dr. Fred Lee of Crittenton Hospital in Rochester, Michigan, is one of the pioneers of PSA screening. He says: "Once you let PSA go up to 4 . . . you've allowed the cancer to grow." And Dr. Lee adds: "A number of us have been lowering 'entrance' PSA to 2. Our center uses a normal PSA of 2. We set our PSA at 2." At Dr. Lee's center, men with a PSA over 2 have an ultrasound examination to look for cancer. Would lowering the upper limit from 4 to 2 result in unnecessary surgery? William J. Catalona, M.D., professor of urology at the Washington University School of Medicine, conducted a study using a PSA cutoff of 2.5. The fear was that a cutoff of 2.5

would result in many inappropriate surgeries. It did not. Dr. Catalona found that 85 percent of radical prostatectomies revealed occult tumors whose grade or volume of disease warranted surgery. How do you know if your PSA is headed toward 4? Dr. Lee says: "We tell patients to *track their PSA.*" The next chapter will show you how.

PSA 1 to 2

There is only a 4 percent chance your PSA will increase to over 4 in the next three years. That's good news and you should feel reassured. What about the 4 percent? There's a full discussion of these rare cases in the appendix.

PSA Less Than 1

There is only a 1 percent chance that your PSA will climb to greater than 4 over the next three years. At less than 1 is where you want your PSA to be. If your value is less than 1, and you're under 50 years of age and at low risk, some doctors recommend less frequent testing until you're 50.

How Often to Test Your PSA

The usual recommendation is a yearly test. If your PSA is rapidly rising or in the normal–high range, consider testing every six months. Many high-powered executives and engineers I know who have high or abnormal PSAs have their PSA measured every three months. Although urologists see this as excessive, these men are paying for their own tests and say that with more points to plot, they can more easily see a trend. If you have a very low score, some experts argue, you could wait two years between tests.

PSA's Success

Rarely in the history of medicine has a simple laboratory test changed the face of a disease, yet that's precisely what the Prostate Specific Antigen test has done. In the old days prostate cancer was considered just a disease of old age. Now it's very much a disease that can affect young, healthy, and virile men, men who never in a million years would have suspected prostate cancer; that is, until the results of their annual physical exam showed an abnormally high level of PSA. The magnitude of new prostate cancer cases diagnosed during the years 1988 to 1995 was unprecedented in the modern history of cancer in the United States.[1] We can thank the PSA test. Cancer was found in hundreds of thousands of men. Their cancers were discovered and removed decades earlier than otherwise would have been possible. As a result, when urologists operate now, it's uncommon to find more advanced cancers. In 1989, when PSA screening began in earnest, 60 percent of cancers removed during surgery were advanced cancers. But after only a year of screening, less than 5 percent of cancers found were advanced. Today, most prostate cancers diagnosed are early-stage and of a much less dangerous grade. Dr. Crawford claims, "Screening has nearly eliminated advanced prostate cancer." Dr. Crawford started the National Prostate Cancer Awareness Week. Johns Hopkins University's Patrick Walsh, M.D., a world leader in prostate cancer surgery, says: "PSA is responsible for the fact that prostate cancer today is not lethal — it's 70 to 80 percent curable." Proponents argue that PSA has been one of the most successful screening tests in history.

WHAT YOU CAN DO NOW

Establish a regular program of PSA and digital rectal exams appropriate to your age and risk.

PSA Testing Tips

• Stick with one company's brand-name test to get consistent results over time. The difference among brands is enough to cause large variations in your PSA level.

• If you're over 50, abstain from sex for at least two days before taking the test. An hour after ejaculation, PSA levels are up to 40 percent higher, but they return to normal within 48 hours. Follow your doctor's instructions carefully to get the most consistent testing results you can.

Tracking PSA

Remember when you were a kid? Was there any better feedback than a great report card? Face it. We love positive feedback, whether it's a great performance review at work or seeing our weight decline on a scale. Well, we can get that same kind of feedback in our program of prostate cancer protection by following our PSA values.

Tracking your PSA values from one year to the next is a unique strategy that allows you to follow the development of a cancer from an extremely early time. Using PSA as your guide, there is the alluring possibility that through an aggressive protective program you could track and virtually stop a microscopic cancer before it becomes uncontrolled cancerous growth. Of course not every cancer can be stopped without surgery, but even then, testing and tracking your PSA will alert you to a malignancy at the earliest possible stage. Imagine if you started tracking your PSA at 0.4 or 1.3 and could contain your PSA so it never got to the danger level? That's the tremendous allure of PSA tracking.

How to Track PSA

Clearly, if you wait for your PSA level to become frankly abnormal, you're waiting too long. That's why thousands of doctors and hundreds of thousands of men look for a trend in their PSA values over time. If you've ever charted stocks or watched a barometer change, you've gotten the sense that following a trend can help you predict what will occur. The way doctors predict what will occur with your PSA is to look for its rate of change. There's a name for that. It's called PSA velocity. If you have your PSA measured regularly and follow it closely over time, it can be the best indication that you are heading into trouble. The Baltimore Longitudinal Aging study found that in men who had a PSA which rose more than 0.75 nanograms per year, the increase was most likely due to cancer. Let's look at real numbers from an actual patient. His values start at an amazingly low value, just 0.6, well off any doctor's radar screen. Look at the results of seven successive tests taken at 6-month intervals. Incredibly, this was not a high-risk patient, yet look at the rise in PSA.

0.6
0.7
0.8
1.1
1.8
2.2
2.4

They're all completely normal values. But look at the increase from 1.1 to 1.8 to 2.2 in just *one* year. That's a jump of 1.1, and that's a tip-off — remember, the Baltimore Longitudinal Aging study found that when the PSA rose more than 0.75 nanograms per year, the increase was more likely due to cancer. Also, look at the jump from 0.8 to 1.1. That's a 27 percent increase, and that is another tip-off. The warning sign doctors look for is an increase of 20 percent from one reading to the next. This patient failed on both counts. Sure enough, the patient had cancer. But it was removed at a very early stage, and his doctor believes the patient's life was saved.

Dr. Peter Carroll of UCSF is following a large group of

men with prostate cancer who have elected to undertake a wait-and-see strategy rather than have surgery or radiation right away. In a new study he has shown that serial PSA levels *are* very strong predictors of who will progress to more serious disease.

Now comes the single most exciting idea in prostate cancer protection. If you can track a PSA as it increases, could you also watch it *decrease?* That's right, using the protective strategies in this book, could you follow your progress by watching your PSA actually decline? Could you watch your PSA back away from the brink? Dr. Catalona says: "There is no downside to treating PSA while it is still low. The theoretical potential is that it may hold the tumor in check and prevent it from increasing." The phrase "treating PSA" simply means that since all you can observe is the PSA level, you take measures to lower the PSA number and assume that by treating the PSA level, you are treating the cancer.

Let's take the case of Robert Yannone. Mr. Yannone was diagnosed with prostate cancer in 1995, when his PSA was 7.5, well into the danger zone. He consulted with one of the best surgeons in the country and with a radiologist from a top cancer center. His treatment of choice? Not surgery, not radiation, but diet. He started eating soy of all kinds, from tofu in his spaghetti to soy yogurt and even tofu ice cream . . . all fat free. He began drinking green tea and eating organic vegetables such as shiitake and portobello mushroooms. His cereals are all organically grown bran cereals. But Robert is not flying blind. He has plotted his PSA level every 6 months since he was diagnosed. The result? "My PSA is now down to 3.9. It's now stabilized at 3.9." You'll recall from the last chapter that 3.9 is a normal reading. "Remember, I'm 75 though, so that's low; and it's still going down. I definitely think it's the diet that has lowered my PSA. The diet, plus the fact that I only eat organic food, so I avoid the preservatives and hormones that they put in nonorganic food." His weight dropped from 156 to 142 (he's five feet nine inches). Like tens of thousands of other American men, Robert gauges his progress with the PSA test.

To many men, the PSA test has become the new cholesterol test. Over the last decade, we as a nation have become obsessed with cholesterol. Cholesterol contents are on every food label, printed on menus, even posted on the nutritional posters in fast-food stores. Talk about our cholesterol test results fills our conversations. We may even reserve bragging rights about achieving a new low cholesterol level for the golf club. Hey! When that level goes down, we're proud! We've made progress. We feel good about ourselves and about our future. Now PSA is poised to become for prostate cancer what cholesterol testing is for heart disease. I hear more and more men talking about their PSA levels and carefully plotting them the way they'd chart their stocks.

How Good Is Following PSA As a Method of Tracking Cancer?

One of the best. PSA is an excellent marker for the effectiveness of standard treatment. After surgery, doctors monitor PSA for evidence of a recurrence. Dr. William Catalano says the PSA test is far more sensitive to changes in tumor size than a rectal exam, biopsy, MRI, CAT scan, or you name it. He says emphatically that if PSA goes down after treatment, it's because there is less tumor producing it. Used to follow tumor treatment, whether by surgery, radiation, or hormonal therapy, a decreased PSA means less tumor. Says Dr. Robert

Krane of Massachusetts General Hospital, "After surgery or hormonal therapy or radiation, PSA is an excellent means of monitoring patients because clinical events (for example, changes in bone scan or a CAT scan) occur much after change in PSA. In other words, the change in PSA will occur *before* you see any growth clinically — that's well accepted." Even doctors who are skeptical of PSA screening still admit it's an excellent test to evaluate the effectiveness of treatment. Appendix Three (page 301) has more on PSA testing used to measure the outcome of standard therapy such as surgery or radiation.

Researchers are now evaluating PSA testing as a means of tracking the effect of diet, lifestyle, and chemoprevention (discussed in the following pages). Dr. Crawford says: "PSA is absolutely a *great* marker for chemoprevention." Dr. Catalano says a decrease in PSA means less tumor even when the treatment is diet. In his patients who already have cancer, diet lowered their PSA for months to years. Preliminary research shows that when men adhere strictly to a prostate cancer diet, they can stabilize and even lower their PSA reading.

WHAT YOU CAN DO NOW

Carefully plot your PSA values. Be sure to read Appendix Three on PSA testing before you start. If you see a rise, consider more frequent testing.

- If your PSA is below 2.0 and the rate of rise is not abnormal, consider the lifestyle program suggested in Part III of this book. Track your progress with PSA. You are the ideal candidate for a prostate cancer protection program.
- If your PSA is between 2.0 and 4.0 and/or your rate of rise

is abnormal, consider further confirmatory testing with your urologist. If you do not have cancer, you, too, are an ideal candidate for a prostate cancer protection program.

- If you have prostate cancer, consider the lifestyle program in this book as an adjunct to standard therapy such as surgery or radiation. Again, 30 percent of men with prostate cancer already take alternative treatments in addition to standard therapy.

- If you have prostate cancer, have a PSA between 4 and 10, and a moderate-grade tumor and are considering diet and lifestyle over surgery, remember that this is an experimental program without known results. If you'd like to undertake this program instead of standard therapy, you should try to do so as part of a clinical trial where you can be followed very carefully. Read the fine print in the appendix before you go further! While this looks like it may be a promising option, you should read what critics say before making your decision.

And remember, if you first choose diet and lifestyle changes, you can always still opt for more aggressive intervention. Take the case of Ivan Flowers, a patient of Dr. William Catalona. He was diagnosed with prostate cancer in January 1999 at age 62. His PSA was 12.8 and his Gleason score was 7. (See page 305 for the complete Gleason scoring system.) He selected diet as his first treatment of choice. "I went on a low-fat diet with lots of vegetables (especially raw broccoli and cauliflower and salads). For meat, I eat only fish and chicken and I've cut out red meat. I eat lots of fruits (apples and oranges and bananas). I eat lots of tofu. I drink a lot of green tea (5 cups a day)." By June, just five months later, his PSA was down to 6.5. "Yes, I *definitely* think that diet has affected the drop in PSA." Even with his success, he did eventually have surgery to be absolutely certain that he was beating his cancer. He knows that PSA is a very good cancer marker, but it's still just a marker. His doctors still didn't know exactly what was happening to his tumor until they removed it. "I will definitely continue eating that diet and taking those supplements. I think that the diet makes me feel more energetic."

Many of the measures in this book have been shown in studies to actually lower PSA — they include lycopene, fiber, genistein, a low-fat diet, stress reduction, lifestyle changes, and all of the drugs in the following section. So track your PSA to see whether the measures are working for you. Use PSA as a benchmark. For more details, see Appendix Three.

In summary, some of prostate cancer's most prominent researchers hope to transform prostate cancer into a chronic disease that might be treated very much like any other chronic disease, with medications and diet and using PSA as a measure of success or failure, much as a cholesterol test is used to measure the effectiveness of cholesterol-lowering therapy.

Chemoprotection

Face it! We're a pill-popping culture. Sure, a great diet and exercise make sense. But what if we could just take a pill? That's what many of us do for heart disease. Sure, lots of us know we should change our lifestyle, but how much easier is it to just take a pill to lower our cholesterol level? Well, why not take a pill to lower our PSA level? That's the idea that hundreds of researchers are now feverishly trying to realize. Across the width and breadth of human cancer research, there is a quest for that wonder pill that can prevent cancer. The field is called chemoprevention, and chemoprevention is a strategy already being used successfully in breast cancer. A drug called tamoxifen has already been approved by the FDA to reduce the risk of breast cancer, which it does by 45 percent. Another drug, called raloxifene, may decrease the risk by up to 79 percent. Pretty impressive results so far. In colon cancer, several promising agents are being tested. In prostate cancer research, scientists are now testing a variety of target drugs. The dream is that one day men could have a simple pill they would take to protect themselves against a prostate cancer ever growing. Some drugs being tested are top secret, such as one being developed by a major Midwestern pharmaceutical company. (No leaks to report!) This chapter will take you through the most interesting chemopreventive agents. While these drugs are all still in the research phase, the vision is that they might turn prostate cancer into a mild, chronic disease that could be treated early with medication rather than later with surgery and radiation. Since it hasn't been shown yet that these drugs will *prevent* a clinical cancer, I'm calling this chapter Chemo*protection*. We'll look at three major strategies: finasteride, exisulind, and PC-SPES. These drugs are already available today for other purposes. That means that as soon as research is conclusive, they will be approved and immediately available to any patient whose physician is willing to prescribe them.

Finasteride

Male sex hormones cause the prostate to grow. When you were a child, your prostate was only the size of a pea. As you became an adolescent, your body started to produce more male sex hormones, which spurred your prostate to grow more quickly to its full adult size and shape — walnut shaped and around an inch and a half long. While you're an adult, your prostate can grow again in middle age when hormonal changes cause further growth. Logically you might ask, "Gee, if sex hormones cause the prostate to grow, couldn't they also cause cancer to grow?" Many researchers believe they do. In fact, Duke University researchers have preliminary evidence which suggests that "the risk of prostate cancer could be linked to the amount of male hormone testosterone circulating in his body as early as puberty or even in utero." Rats get prostate cancer after being given testosterone over prolonged periods of time. The next logical question is this: If hormones cause prostate cancer to grow, isn't there some way of blocking those hormones and protecting yourself against the growth of a prostate cancer? Many researchers believe the answer is yes.

First let's start by understanding two key male sex hormones, testesterone and dihydrotestosterone (DHT), and their possible role in prostate cancer. Male sex hormones as a group are referred to as androgens.

Testosterone

Testosterone is the foremost male sex hormone because it's responsible for a man's "virility," that is, his secondary sex characteristics such as a deep voice or body hair or even fertility. The testicles make about 95 percent of a man's testosterone. Once in the prostate, testosterone has little effect. To stimulate the prostate, it must first be converted to another hormone called DHT (dihydrotestosterone), which is the active form of testosterone in the prostate.

DHT

DHT is quite simply the most powerful male hormone in the body, two to ten times more powerful than testosterone. But here's why DHT is so critical to prostate cancer. DHT attaches to a receptor deep in the cell called an androgen nuclear receptor. This is the same lock-and-key principle we looked at in the chapter on fats. Once the key and lock match, it's as if a switch were turned, like putting a key into your car's ignition and starting the engine. The analogy fits here because once DHT locks onto a receptor deep within the cell in its nucleus, it increases the growth of prostate cells.

So how much DHT do you have in your prostate? You might think that depends on the amount of testosterone your body makes. That's not the case. Your individual level of DHT is governed by an enzyme called 5 alpha-reductase, and that differs substantially from man to man. An enzyme drives a chemical reaction, making it go faster than it would without the enzyme. Think of the enzyme as a catalyst. The enzyme 5 alpha-reductase converts testosterone into dihydrotestosterone (DHT). How much 5 alpha-reductase do you have? You can see by the amount of body hair you have.

Why? 5 alpha-reductase is also found in the skin. Men with more 5 alpha-reductase have more local sex hormone stimulation in the skin. The result can be seen in the increased growth of body hair and beard and moustache, but, paradoxically, more baldness on the head. The key to remember is that 5 alpha-reductase determines how much DHT you have in your prostate. There's more detail on DHT in Appendix Two.

If male sex hormones could increase the risk of cancer, could blocking them decrease the risk? We already know that blocking the effects of these hormones works as a treatment in some men with advanced prostate cancer. To test the idea that DHT is involved in the growth of prostate cancer, the National Cancer Institute is using a drug to block the production and subsequent effect of DHT on the prostate. The drug being tested for prostate cancer is called finasteride.

Finasteride is manufactured by the drug company Merck. It's already in widespread usage under the trade name Proscar as a treatment for benign prostatic hypertrophy (BPH) and under the trade name Propecia for the treatment of male pattern baldness. Here's how it works. Finasteride blocks the conversion of testosterone to the much stronger DHT that promotes prostate growth. (Finasteride resembles the hormone testosterone. When the enzyme 5 alpha-reductase goes looking for testosterone, it finds finasteride instead. Because finasteride has a slightly higher chemical binding capacity than testosterone, finasteride has a better shot at attaching to 5 alpha-reductase enzyme than testosterone. Now 5 alpha-reductase can't convert real testosterone to DHT because the enzyme is blocked by finasteride. The bottom line is that finasteride should decrease the amount of DHT in the prostate.)

Researchers are testing whether finasteride might prevent

prostate cancer for a number of reasons. Finasteride did prevent prostate cancer in one Japanese study with rats. Doctors
also noticed that patients taking finasteride to treat BPH have
low PSA readings — and since the PSA level is one indicator
for cancer, researchers wanted to inquire whether a lower
PSA means less cancer.

Finasteride Study Specifics

In November 1993, the NCI started the finasteride trial,
called the Prostate Cancer Prevention Trial. In this study, researchers are following 18,000 healthy men for seven years.
Volunteers are from 222 sites in the U.S. and Canada. It took
researchers three years to get 18,000 men, so the last men will
be examined in 2003. Each man was 55 years of age or older
at the time of entry; the median age at entry was 62. Half the
men are taking daily pills of finasteride, and half are taking
placebos. The study is double blind, which means that neither
the participants nor the doctors will know who's taking finasteride until the end of the trial. For seven years each man
is followed and screened annually with a PSA test and a digital rectal exam; and at the end, all will be biopsied. The study
is aimed at answering three questions: a) does finasteride
lower the risk of getting prostate cancer? b) does finasteride
lower the risk of having BPH? and c) does looking at PSA velocity, in other words, year-to-year PSA level, improve the accuracy of prostate cancer diagnosis?

Although the verdict on finasteride and prostate cancer is
still not in, some researchers have misgivings about the drug;
but researchers at the NCI think many of these misgivings ill
placed. The appendix presents both sides of the argument.

Other Uses of Finasteride

BPH: BPH is a common condition that begins in middle age when a man's prostate becomes enlarged enough to make urinating difficult. By reducing the amount of DHT, finasteride slows prostate growth. In fact, over time finasteride shrinks the enlarged prostate.

Male pattern balding: Finasteride is also prescribed to balding men because it lowers the androgenic stimulation to their skin, so hair grows back on their heads, while at the same time they lose some body hair. The FDA has approved finasteride for both BPH and male pattern balding. Should finasteride be proved to prevent prostate cancer, it could become a blockbuster drug for its nearly universal appeal to middle-aged men: its ability to help prevent baldness, BPH, and prostate cancer. If you currently take finasteride, see page 294 for special guidelines you'll need to track your PSA, since the drug does alter PSA levels.

Lowering Testosterone Levels

See Appendix Two for drugs and supplements that affect testosterone. The big question most men ask is, "Gee, if I lower my testosterone level, will it affect my *virility?*" Says Ronald Ross, M.D., of the University of Southern California, "We're talking about variations in the normal testosterone ranges; that wouldn't affect virility. But a difference that could be small and not affect virility may make a huge difference in prostate cancer risk over long periods of time."

Exisulind

Exisulind is a drug you might one day take every morning, just like a vitamin, in order to prevent prostate cancer. In very preliminary tests, it has already been shown to stabilize PSA or even to lower PSA.

Exisulind does kill prostate cancer cells. When scientists took prostate cancer cells and put them in a dish and added exisulind, they noticed a much greater cell death than with cells that were not treated with exisulind. And Erik Goluboff, M.D., of Columbia University, has shown in animal studies that exisulind prevents the growth of prostate cancer in live animals. Dr. Goluboff took human prostate cancer cells and injected them into mice with no immune systems. He divided the mice into three groups. The first group was mice who ate regular food, and the result was that their tumors quadrupled in size in 4 weeks! The second group consisted of mice who got food supplemented with exisulind, and their tumors grew 25 percent in 4 weeks. The third group had mice who got food supplemented with a much higher dose of exisulind, and their tumors grew 18 percent in 4 weeks.

Dr. Goluboff recently completed a human trial testing exisulind for management of recurrent prostate cancer. Based on his work and the safety profile from colon cancer studies that showed exisulind is well tolerated, he led a multicentered, double-blind, randomized, placebo-controlled phase III clinical trial, the gold standard for clinical trials. There were 90 patients in the trial, which was conducted at UCLA, at Columbia, in Pittsburgh, and in Florida. At each center, half of the patients took the drug and half did not, and they didn't know whether they were receiving the drug or the placebo. The interim analysis at 6 months, which was the halfway point of the study, showed that men who were on the drug had a leveling of their PSA, whereas men not taking exisulind had a PSA that was still rising exponentially. The study was recently completed, and a preliminary analysis indicates that the final results confirm the observations made at the 6-month interim. All of the patients in the study had had prostatectomies. After the operation, their doctors observed a rapid increase in PSA. That means that there was cancer still in their bodies and it was growing at a rapid pace, which is why they were admitted to the study. Says Dr. Goluboff, "PSA levels going up indicates growing disease. All patients in the trial were chosen because their PSA levels had gone up quickly after their prostatectomy, so we treated them to slow their rise of PSA so they don't get metastasis. If you've had your prostate removed for cancer, and your PSA goes up, then that's an indication that you have cancer; so if you treat PSA and see that it's rising very slowly, then you know the cancer cells are not growing and dividing quickly . . . in essence the person is cured."

Cell Pathways is producing exisulind. At this point, the drug is still at research stages, so there are no recommendations by professional organizations, but you should follow closely the outcomes of the human trials, as they might revolutionize prostate cancer prevention and treatment.

PC-SPES

PC-SPES, many think, is the hottest new sensation in prostate cancer treatment. But be warned that it is also hotly controversial. What you'll read here is a fair account of what it does and why you may or may not want to take it . . . yet. PC-SPES stands for Prostate Cancer Hope. "Spes" is the Latin word for "hope" . . . as you'll remember from those painful days in high school. PC-SPES is made of 8 different herbs — one American herb and 7 Chinese herbs. PC-SPES has a hodgepodge of different actions, some quite specific, others rather vague.

The Birth of PC-SPES

Sophie Chen, Ph.D., is the mother of PC-SPES. She is director of NovaSpes Research Laboratory and research associate professor at New York Medical College. She realized the limitations of developing a single chemical to treat a chronic disease. In fact, in most cancer treatments, multiple agents are used to get the best effect. In 1987, Dr. Chen started her own research on a combination therapy that would include different herbs for prostate cancer. She worked in collaboration with Professor Xu-Hui Wang, an herbal medical doctor and director of the Shanghai Medical University for Herbal Medicine in China. Dr. Wang comes from five generations of medical practitioners in China. His great-grandfather worked with the Chinese emperor and so he has secret family recipes. His father had an M.D. from Germany — so Dr. Wang knows the medical traditions of both the West and the East.

Dr. Chen took Dr. Wang's recipes, changed some of the ingredients, and designed experiments to test them in vitro (in lab) and in vivo (in animals). She also examined the chemical content of each herb to understand how it worked. Now here's where luck intervened. At the time she was developing a combination therapy for cancer, a relative of Dr. Chen's developed terminal prostate cancer, and she tried to customize the recipes for him. She and Dr. Wang took a biopsy from the patient and grew his sample tumors in mice to study and test them with herbal combinations. In 1991–1992 Dr. Chen and Dr. Wang finally developed PC-SPES based on the relative's tumor. When the patient started treatment, the cancer had metastasized to his rib and pelvic bone. In other words, it was the worst late-stage prostate cancer you could have. To their astonishment, with PC-SPES he went into remission within 6 months. Today, seven years later, he is in total remission and good physical condition. Although this case is just one anecdote, PC-SPES, as we'll see, has been used with success since that time.

PC-SPES has two roles. First, proponents say, it's enjoying enormous success in treatment of advanced prostate cancer. Second, PC-SPES is being analyzed as a potential preventive treatment. For the purposes of this book, what's most remarkable about PC-SPES is that it improves PSA for the majority of patients. "There's more than a 50 percent reduction in PSA in 3 months," says Dr. Chen. PC-SPES is included here because of its remarkable ability to lower PSA and because it is being used in current prevention trials.

How Does PC-SPES Work?

PC-SPES is a holistic approach that seeks to attack a cancer in several important ways. The holistic approach claims that combination medicine is better than the single-bullet approach. "Combination" means combining either different herbs or different synthetic compounds or combining natural and synthetic compounds. "Holistic" means thinking of the whole body — if you kill cancer cells, you still want to take into consideration the rest of the body (that's why immune enhancement is important as a buffer to protect against problems elsewhere in the body). Says Dr. Chen: "Especially for the treatment of cancer, the holistic approach is important. I only see a solution to treating cancer if there's a combination approach. The magic bullet [i.e., a single drug] approach is very unlikely because of the heterogenous population of cancer cells and the fact that the body has several pathways through which the cancer can come back. In 30 years we've seen no great improvement for advanced-stage patients' outcome because we've been using the magic-bullet approach."

Holistic drugs usually contain active compounds to kill cancer cells, compounds to enhance the immune system, and specialized drug-carrier systems that help to target only cancer cells.

The herbs in PC-SPES contain 4 different kinds of agents:

- anticancer herbs
- anti-inflammatory herbs
- antiviral herbs
- immune enhancement herbs

"The combination is very synergistic, very holistic," says Dr. Chen. "Combined, these herbs kill cancer cells, reduce the cancer genes, reduce inflammation, reduce the androgen receptor, and enhance the immune system." For a full list of the ingredients, see Appendix Two.

Eric Small, M.D., of UC San Francisco, says there is no question that some of the anticancer effects of PC-SPES are estrogenic. In other words, one way that cancer cells are tamed by PC-SPES is through its estrogen-like effect. Estrogen is known to be active against advanced prostate cancer that is still sensitive to hormones. The rationale for hormone therapy is that it deprives the cancer cells of androgens, or male sex hormones. Since those androgen hormones drive cancer growth, depriving cancer cells of them slows, stops, or even reverses the growth of the cancer . . . for months to years. The question is, is this hormone effect PC-SPES's only really important drug-like quality? Dr. Small recently reported that PC-SPES is also effective for hormone-insensitive patients, which might indicate that PC-SPES is not just an herbal estrogen.

Side Effects

The main side effects of PC-SPES come from its role as an estrogen. The mild estrogenic-seeming side effects are nipple tenderness, some breast enlargement (in many men this is quite significant), and a decrease in libido. In one study, 0.5 percent of patients reported diarrhea, but diarrhea and breast tenderness are dependent on dosage, Dr. Chen thinks. The dosage was 9 capsules per day (3 capsules three times a day). Each capsule was 320 milligrams. There have also been anecdotal reports of heart attacks.

About 2 percent of patients on PC-SPES showed blood-clotting problems. Of the 2,000 patients on the drug, one patient died of a stroke. But Dr. Chen points out that both of his parents had died of a stroke and that he had had hypertension and also blood-coagulation problems.

Standardization

Dr. Chen is performing quality control by chemical analysis and by biological assay. The animal assay to test toxicity shows that PC-SPES is 25 times less toxic than aspirin, which is important since the World Health Organization (WHO) has a toxicity guideline requiring supplements to be 5 times safer than aspirin.

Human Studies

PC-SPES sounds great, but how do we know it works? There have been three successful clinical studies on PC-SPES: one in Germany and two at the University of California at San Francisco. These are all in patients who already have prostate cancer. There are several publications on these clinical studies of PC-SPES. The studies include prostate cancer patients from early stage to terminal stage. In all groups, patients seem to respond to PC-SPES with PSA reduction of higher than 50 percent, tumor volume decrease of more than 50 percent, and improvement in quality of life. The appendix has the details of all three studies.

Advantages of PC-SPES over Traditional Therapy

Advocates say that PC-SPES is superior to chemotherapy and hormone therapy because of the much better quality of life it offers. Here's why.

• Advantages over chemotherapy: no hair loss or reduced quality-of-life side effects.

• Advantages over hormone therapy: no muscle loss, osteoporosis, or memory loss due to hormone therapy.

What the Experts Say

Since the evolution of PC-SPES as a preventive treatment is still unproved, many top specialists are less than enthusiastic about it. If you are seriously considering taking PC-SPES, be sure to read in the appendix their warnings about it.

The bottom line: Most experts interviewed seemed to agree that PC-SPES does work like an estrogen, like hormonal treatment. The question is whether it is any better — or worse — than conventional treatment, or if it has additional important effects.

Who Should Consider Taking PC-SPES?

PC-SPES is in clinical use to treat patients with advanced prostate cancer. Dr. Chen is also working on a lower-potency PC-SPES supplement for prevention. This supplement would be taken as one takes a vitamin; and it would be taken by younger men at high risk (e.g., with a family history of prostate cancer), or by men over 50. Currently, because of the estrogen-like actions, few men with a normal PSA would consider taking it. If you have a high PSA and want to take PC-SPES, be sure you are being observed as part of a clinical trial, and be wary that a drop in PSA, should you have one, may not mean that you are beating the tumor.

Let's take a look at a real case history. Harry Pinchot was diagnosed with metastatic prostate cancer. Androgen-deprivation therapy and the drug thalidomide failed him after 11 or 12 months. Here's what PC-SPES has done for him:

> I'm the longest survivor of post-hormone therapy on PC-SPES. Usually when you fail hormone therapy you're on the down slope. You're a short-timer. If you do hormone therapy and that fails, then they do a little chemotherapy and that's it. We had beautiful results with PC-SPES. I have 36 months of posthormone therapy and postchemotherapy on PC-SPES. I feel compelled to teach people. My current PSA is 0.031. When it got to 0.06, my doctor and I increased the PC-SPES dose to lower PSA, and it did lower it.

How to Take PC-SPES

PC-SPES is available in capsules. You should take it only under a doctor's supervision. It's best taken before eating, although it can be taken with or without food. The dose is dependent on use, with the higher doses reserved for those with prostate cancer.

Where to Buy PC-SPES

While on PC-SPES, you'll need to be monitored by a doctor; so you'll also need a doctor's recommendation to buy the supplement. PC-SPES is now being sold through some doctors and health care professionals and nature pharmacies. If you have a doctor's recommendation, you can also directly call the company that produces it, Botaniclab, in California (714-524-5533). In any case, you'll have to pay for it yourself. Since PC-SPES is now being sold as a nutritional supplement and not as a drug, it's not under the preview of the FDA. And as long as PC-SPES does not have FDA approval, no insurance company will cover it. It will cost you an average of $252 per month. Since the supplement is not a prescription drug, it's also not being used by hospitals.

Conclusion

There is a strong rivalry between advocates of diet versus advocates of drugs. A race is on between the two schools . . . which will be the first to prove it can protect you from prostate cancer? Fortunately, it's a race that can only benefit us as men. The one downside of the pill is that while you may be spared from prostate cancer, you may continue many of the faulty diet and lifestyle habits that could bring on other diseases associated with the Western diet — for example, diabetes and obesity. That makes me a strong believer in the school that promotes diet and lifestyle. Keep in mind that if your risk is high, you could end up doing both! As you'll see in the personal accounts of men on a prostate cancer protection plan, most combine diet, exercise, and stress management with drugs and standard therapy.

Surgery

I sat with a group of prostate cancer patients. Each of them had seriously considered standard surgical treatment for his cancer. After carefully weighing all the alternatives, they had all chosen to treat their cancer, under the very close supervision of their doctors, with a rigorous diet and lifestyle program. I asked them and their wives what was the number one reason they had avoided surgery. They giggled, smiled, and said "*sex.*" What they feared most about surgery was an end to a happy and healthy sex life. Another group of prostate cancer survivors met. Each person had had a complete surgical removal of his prostate performed within the previous year. These men appeared morose, even depressed. Many complained of the need to wear diapers. Months after the operation, many no longer had any sex life at all. Those who had recovered talked about what surgeons refer to as a "stuffable erection," but not a solid, firm one. One patient volunteered that he'd trade five great years for fifteen impotent ones. Given a second chance, he'd never do the operation again.

Many prostate cancer survivors claim that the real rates of impotence and incontinence can be far higher than you hear in the media. For instance, while 86 percent of men may remain potent after the operation in the best of hands, the average rate of impotence is a little less than *fifty* percent! I spoke with a childhood friend of mine who had had surgery at a top Harvard hospital but still remained incontinent and impotent a year later. He had been assured the nerves that innervate the penis would be spared and that he would remain continent and potent, but that's not what happened. For that reason diet, nutritional therapy, exercise, stress control, chemoprevention, and supplements are gaining enthusiasm and support. Proponents of the lifestyle approach point out that there is no guarantee that surgery will cure you, nor are there any rigorous long-term studies that prove surgery saves lives. Experts are seeking another alternative, and that is perfect surgery — surgery that will cure you *and* leave you potent.

For decades, many surgeons assumed the nerves that control potency were *in* the prostate itself, so that there was no alternative but to cut them as the prostate was removed. In the hundreds of years of dissecting human cadavers, no one had ever actually found them. Patrick C. Walsh, M.D, chairman of the famous Johns Hopkins Department of Urology, took up the challenge. Through meticulous and painstaking work, he and his colleagues located the nerves. To his great surprise and delight, they were outside the prostate. Why not, he thought, remove the prostate and spare the nerves that control potency and urinary continence? That's exactly what he did in what is now called a "nerve-sparing" operation. Although he is too modest to allow the procedure to be named after him, it's commonly called "the Walsh procedure."

The Walsh procedure, however, is not perfect. Fourteen percent of men may still become impotent. When I asked Dr. Walsh about this in his office one afternoon, rather than answering defensively, there was a gleam in his eye. He hinted that a nearly perfect operation was in the offing. He had carefully and painstakingly reviewed the videotapes of the nerve-sparing procedures that he had done. He found some almost trivial variations in the procedures. These tiny variations could account for the loss of potency or delayed recovery of some patients. For instance, a sheath is cut during the operation. Afterwards, it seems natural to pull the two edges of the sheath together so it will heal as a single sheath. However, the stress of pulling the two sides together may put excess stress on the nerves, prolonging recovery. Sure enough, when he looked at the patients with minor imperfections in the surgery, they were the ones having problems. Not big problems, but nonetheless, slower recovery and "stuffable" erections.

Although many other centers of excellence offer the operation, as do doctors in private practice, there are also surgeons who have not mastered the technique. That's why if you consider the procedure, be sure you know exactly what kind of results your surgeon gets. You'll want potency rates in excess of 80 percent. Many surgeons, including Dr. Walsh, keep statistics so that their patients have an objective way of comparing results.

Measuring Outcomes

How do you know what kind of result you will get from surgery? When you choose a surgeon, be sure that the medical center he or she operates from has superior outcomes as well. The best guarantee is going to a center of excellence that keeps a record of the actual outcomes of surgery. That way you know what the track record is. For instance, the University of California at San Francisco compared its results to a national dataset of patients and found much better than average outcomes, reports urologist-in-chief Peter Carroll, M.D.

Outcomes are defined generally by five variables:

- cancer stage and grade
- patient age and general health, including potency status
- type of treatment: surgery, radiation, or a combination of both

- skill of the surgeon
- method of outcome assessment: e.g., physician versus patient reporting, and qualitative versus quantitative results

Experts can control for these variables to compare one institution to another. For instance, if one institution sees much older, sicker patients with more advanced disease, their results may be poorer. But by controlling for these differences, they can make a fair comparison. You're already ahead of the game if you go to an institution that measures outcomes. The vast majority of patients' outcomes are never measured, says Dr. Carroll.

One note of caution: Not every man can have a nerve-sparing operation. There are those patients whose tumors are so close to the nerves that there is no alternative but to cut through them. Still, there is new hope even for them.

New Hope

Even for men who've had a prostatectomy and become impotent, or who are facing a prostatectomy in which the potency nerves *must* be cut, hope is on the horizon. Doctors at Baylor College and M.D. Anderson Cancer Center in Houston are now experimenting with a new technique to actually transplant nerves from the leg to restore potency in men who would otherwise become impotent after prostate surgery — this procedure must be done at the time of surgery, not after. For others, who still have some nerve function intact after surgery, the drug Viagra has been a godsend. If you can't take Viagra or don't like the side effects, there's the Caverject system. Caverject is a drug that a man injects into his penis to achieve erection. Although Caverject involves an injection with a very small needle, most men find the pain negligible and the result terrific. In fact, some men who started with Caverject and then tried Viagra have returned to Caverject.

When to Consider Surgery

The most important concern is this: at what point does a cancer go from curable to incurable? You clearly don't want to wait so long that you allow your cancer to become incurable. No one can tell you when that point is, which is why, in your PSA-tracking program, you should keep an open mind about surgery. For instance, nearly 40 percent of men in a watchful-waiting program eventually opted for surgery. Dr. Carroll, who studied them, found that by waiting most did not compromise their chances of a cure. Dr. William Catalona, as well, has many patients who first controlled their disease with diet and then opted for surgery. Take as an example George Salazar, a patient of Dr. Catalona's. When he was diagnosed, he changed his diet. This is what he chose to do: He began drinking 3 to 4 cups a day of green tea and started taking lycopene extract (15 milligrams twice a day). He binged on tomatoes, drinking 2 to 3 glasses of tomato juice a day and having plenty of tomatoes in salads and cooked dishes. He took vitamin E (400 IU a day) and other antioxidants, drank orange juice, and ate lots of fruits and vegetables. He stayed away from red meat. The result? His PSA dropped from 7.6 to 4.1 in a little over two months — an amazing result. He says, "I have my high hopes that it was because of diet." Still, he elected to have surgery *and* to continue the diet.

There are also other alternatives to surgery for men who have cancer and have advanced disease or cannot undergo surgery — for example radioactive implants and radiation. While these are good choices for some men, they are beyond the scope of this book. I'd strongly recommend visiting the

CaP CURE Web site (www.capcure.org) and reading the following books, as they have clear and excellent presentations:

> Patrick C. Walsh, M.D., and Janet Farrar Worthington,
> *The Prostate: A Guide for Men and the Women Who
> Love Them* (Baltimore: Johns Hopkins University
> Press, 1995), and Joseph E. Oesterling, M.D., and
> Mark A. Moyad, M.P.H, *The ABCs of Prostate
> Cancer: The Book That Could Save Your Life*
> (Lanham, Md.: Madison Books, 1997).

To be perfectly clear, surgery still has a very prominent place in the treatment of prostate cancer. This book is not advocating that you treat yourself with diet or supplements rather than undergoing proven treatment if you have been diagnosed with prostate cancer. However, if after considering all the data, you and your doctor do elect to "wait and see" rather than have surgery, an aggressive lifestyle program is an excellent adjunct. I advise, however, very careful, frequent, and close observation if you choose to delay surgery. Many experts believe that you can begin to see when you are getting into trouble by following a rise in PSA or growth as seen on scans of the prostate, so you can have the operation before it's too late, but they have no proof that this is true. Other equally qualified experts believe that the current testing techniques are not accurate enough to be sure that your cancer is not growing or spreading. This book is best used to protect yourself from prostate cancer *before* you develop a clinical cancer. Should you be diagnosed with prostate cancer, you should seriously consider standard treatment, including surgery. If you undertake surgery, follow the principles in this chapter to get the lowest complication rate possible.

Part Five

Close

This is a wonderfully exciting time in prostate cancer research. Many great minds and terrific laboratories, foundations, clinics, and university medical centers have joined the race to find a cure. They have also joined a race to prevent prostate cancer. You stand to benefit enormously by what you have learned in this book and by continuing to follow the research. The Association for the Cure of Cancer of the Prostate (CaP CURE) has an excellent Web site that will allow you to follow these developments — www.capcure.org. You can also call CaP CURE at 800-757-2873 to receive their latest publication on prostate cancer.

I've adopted the program in this book and feel the best I ever have, and I'm not alone. Dr. Charles Myers of the University of Virginia is a top prostate cancer specialist whose work is quoted throughout this book. Ironically, he is battling prostate cancer himself and is now eating a low-fat diet that incorporates many of the terrific foods discussed in this book. "It may sound as though this decreases your pleasure in life but, in fact, you'll feel so much better that you won't want to go back to your old ways of eating. I've had my patients say that to me, and now I've experienced it myself." For men like himself with prostate cancer, he adds: "If a man already has prostate cancer, he should be thinking about everything he can do to stack the cards in his favor; and diet is *one* thing he can control."

This book offers an outstanding lifestyle that will help you overcome the afflictions the Western diet and lifestyle impose on us: diabetes, heart disease, cancers, obesity, stress. Be reassured that on the way to far better health, you are doing the most you can to protect yourself against prostate cancer. This program is remarkably similar to an ideal breast cancer prevention plan, so your whole family can enjoy the new way of life. Good luck.

Personal Programs

Hey, nice suggestions, Dr. Bob, but does anybody really eat the foods or practice the lifestyle programs in this book? You bet! Thousands of men. Each of them constructs his own unique program. Let's see how real men are using all the elements in this book. Some already have prostate cancer and are trying to prevent a recurrence or even trying to treat their disease with lifestyle changes. For each of these men, you'll find a personal cancer history and an actual diet. I'd like to thank each man for being brave enough to tell his own personal story and for sharing what he does as a great example for the rest of us. This book has neat and clean divisions into diet, lifestyle, chemo-protection, and surgery, but in the real world, men take every shot they can at beating this disease. There is no dividing line for them between traditional and alternative treatments. Whatever works is best. Some men have used every single measure in this book — foods, diet, stress reduction, lifestyle, drugs, surgery, supplements — you name it! PSA measurement is often how they judge success. You'll find each of them has a tremendous knowledge of medicine and nutrition. Each one has taken a bold and courageous stand against prostate cancer. Here are their stories in their own words.

Mike Milken, Founder, CaP CURE

My Cancer History

I was 46 years old when I was diagnosed. It was 1993. I had a routine physical and a digital rectal exam by an internist, who said I was fine. I was taking blood tests and the doctor said I was in fantastic condition. I said, "Take my PSA," and he said, "Why? You're young." I said, "Take it anyway." One of my closest friends, Steve Ross, chairman of Time Warner, had just died of prostate cancer. The internist took a blood test and called me a few weeks later and said, "You're in great health, but there must be a mistake with your PSA because it came back 24." I took a blood test that day, and it came back again at around 24. A urologist gave me another digital rectal exam and said I had a mass. My Gleasons were 8 and 9. [See the table in Appendix Three for an explanation of the Gleason scoring system.] I had advanced cancer, and every single biopsy was found positive for cancer. I took an MRI and CAT scans. There was cancer in my lymph nodes. Some of my lymph nodes were almost 50 to 100 percent enlarged. I was getting more and more negative news, until I took a bone scan and they said my bones had not been touched.

I then visited with several scientists. I talked to as many people as I could. I visited Chinese chi doctors. I moved a doctor who practices Indian medicine into my home.

My Western medicine treatment consisted of hormone therapy (flutamide and leuprolide) and radiation therapy. My PSA went to 0 in 4 to 5 months of hormone therapy. Then, 8 months later, I started radiation therapy, which lasted around 3 months.

When I was diagnosed, I immediately changed my diet and lifestyle. I did aromatherapy, massage therapy, yoga, and meditation, and significantly changed my diet. I stopped eating except for steamed vegetables and fruits. I tried to go to the beach and sat on the beach and visited gardens. I listened to classical music and other types of music. As soon as I could, I took up a regular workout routine. I worked out in the gym 3 times a week for an hour — aerobic exercise and weight training for an hour. Also, a couple of times a week I played tennis and other recreational sports.

I still do the hormone therapy. I'm still on flutamide and leuprolide.

I still have my regular workout routine.

I do yoga and meditation — on average, combined, 30 to 45 minutes per day.

My Diet Today

Everything I eat today is from my two cookbooks, so when I refer to a recipe, it's a recipe from those cookbooks. The recipes are all very healthy. We've even developed a recipe for glazed doughnuts and Philadelphia cheese steaks (it was the first time I'd had cheese steaks in 25 years!). We have taken these foods to kids in the inner cities, and they couldn't tell the difference.

- Breakfast: Between 8 and 10 in the morning I have a soy shake. I put brewed green tea and 3 to 4 tablets of green tea, juice (orange or apple), fruits (all kinds, with lots of berries), zest of oranges and lemons, and soy powder (3 scoops) into my shake. I might have 2 of those shakes a day. I have well over 100 grams of soy protein a day.
- I might then have granola, fruit, pancakes, or waffles. Some days I just have a shake. The granola, pancakes, and waffles are all from the cookbooks. I love my nonfat potato pancakes.
- Lunch: I'll have a soup from my cookbooks. I'll eat Cuban sandwiches with tofu and salami (also made from soy) and soy cheeses. I'll have tofu hot dogs, or a chef salad, or southwestern salad, or Caesar salad (I have 3 or 4 Caesar

salads a week). Or I'll enjoy spaghetti, pizza, lasagne —
again, all from my cookbooks.

- Dinner: For dinner, I'll have any of those foods I also men-
tioned for lunch.
- I must eat more than a dozen fruits and vegetables a day.
The dishes I eat have plenty of garlic, onions, and scallions.
- I take 100 to 200 mcg of selenium a day; I put it in my soy
drink.
- I take 500 to 800 IU of vitamin E a day, also in my soy
drink.

My diet is now the same as when I was a kid, but made
with healthy ingredients and lots of soy.

Today my PSA is 0. I attribute that to the hormones that
I still take, the radiation I had when I was diagnosed, my
mental attitude, exercise, aromatherapy, massage therapy,
yoga, and diet.

We have strived to leave our children with a country free
from debt, yet we are burdening them with massive medical
costs associated with an aging population and ever-increasing
rates of cancer.

We have strived to leave our children with a world that cel-
ebrates and cherishes the sanctity of a single human life, yet we
are unwilling to make the financial and moral commitments
necessary to lift the burden of cancer from the next generation.

Through sins of omission as well as commission, we have
created a world where one in five children will have their lives
cut short by cancer. This is too great a burden to leave to our
children and grandchildren.

For those children and the children of future generations,
let us find a cure for cancer. Let us do it now. Let us choose life.

Dr. Charles Myers

My Cancer History

I went in for my first screening exam in February 1999, at age
55. The urologist said, "There's a nodule," so she did a
biopsy and it was positive and my PSA was 20. I had a Gleason score of 7. So the first thing was to see if the cancer was
still localized or whether it had metastasized; exams showed
that it hadn't metastasized. But statistically, it was likely that
the cancer had broken through the capsule of the prostate
gland. That ruled out surgery; but radiation therapy can ra-
diate and treat the cancer around the prostate, too, and the
area outside the prostate in the surrounding tissues. That's
why I chose radiation therapy. Hormonal therapy is important because it makes the radiation more effective. When cancer cells are faced with both hormonal and radiation therapy
it's a double hit, and that increases tumor kill.

My diagnosis was on February 8. By early April, I knew
what I was dealing with. Starting in February, I began the
hormone therapy — I took Lupron [leuprolide], which turns
off the production of testosterone in the testes, and Casodex
[bicalutamide], which prevents testosterone from being produced by the adrenal gland, and Proscar [finasteride], which
prevents the conversion of testosterone into DHT. In May I
started the radiation therapy, and that went on for one
month. In June I rested. On July 8, I had radioactive seeds
placed in my prostate gland.

My Diet Today

• As soon as I had the diagnosis, I went on the diet I knew I
  needed to be on — a vegan (no animal or dairy products),

low-fat diet. The fat in my diet is at 10 to 15 percent. I eat lots of fresh fruits and vegetables, grains and beans, and soy products (nonfat soymilk, miso to flavor soups, et cetera, roasted soy nuts, soybeans cooked in soups and stews, black soybeans, edamame). I don't care much for tofu. I eat lots of salads, greens (for example, rapini, an Italian broccoli-like vegetable with a bitter flavor that we cook with garlic), a lot of winter squash, artichokes, broccoli, and asparagus. We have a vegetable garden and we grow tomatoes and can them. I also drink V-8, which I love.

- After radiation you can't drink tea and coffee because they make your bladder burn. Now that the radiation side effects are subsiding, I can drink some green tea (one cup in the morning).

- Olive oil is the one fat that is safe.

- As for supplements, I take vitamin E (400 IU per day) and selenium (200 mcg of selenium yeast per day). In the first few months after the seeds were implanted, I used saw palmetto to help reduce the swelling of the prostate gland, 2 capsules twice a day. Saw palmetto is the berry of the saw palmetto plant, which grows along the Atlantic coastal plain. It acts as an anti-inflammatory and reduces swelling of the prostate; it is regularly used for BPH. For pain relief I took Celebrex (celecoxib). I take no other supplements.

- I eat a little bit of dark chocolate, which adds some sunlight without adding a great risk. Dark chocolate has stearic acid, which we think is good. Chocolate is made of cocoa powder and cocoa butter. Cocoa powder has the same polyphenols found in green tea but in higher concentration. The cocoa butter is the fat but it's got stearic acid in it, and stearic acid might not be as dangerous as we think. (Stearic acid is one fat that does not increase the risk of heart disease.) A paper published by Dr. Giovannucci on the Physicians' Health Study showed that the physicians with the most stearic acid in their blood had a 70 percent reduction in their risk of metastatic prostate cancer. When I saw that, I couldn't imagine where they got their stearic acid, and then I found it was probably partly from chocolate. We went back to the lab and tested stearic acid and found that it *does* kill prostate cancer cells in test tubes.

There is kosher chocolate without dairy. Ghirardelli also makes a chocolate candy bar without milk fat. Hershey's makes a cocoa powder without fat.

Bob Each

My Cancer History

I was diagnosed with prostate cancer on November 15, 1995, at 11 A.M. It was one of the worst moments of my life. I had extremely advanced disease. My Gleason scores were 8 and 9. My PSA was in the 100s — I was too dumb to get the precise number. I had between 8 and 12 bone metastases — rib, spine, femur, hips. Two weeks later I went for a second opinion and was told I had 6 months to 3 years to live. With that information I tried to scour the earth for ideas.

I have a daughter with a degree in nutrition, and she was the first to say nutrition was of benefit. Some literature she gave me said that if you ate a diet of less than 20 percent fat, it would reduce rate of growth. Then I went to an oncologist in the L.A. area who reinforced the diet concept. He also gave me more drugs.

Over the years, I have become more strict about my diet, and I've used some alternative therapies. At first I did hormone therapy — it was the only therapy available. Hormone therapy worked fairly well. After a year of hormone therapy my PSA was 4; then I started taking PC-SPES. My PSA has decreased over the years and is now 0.151, which I am pleased with.

Now my only form of therapy is diet and PC-SPES. I take nine capsules a day of PC-SPES, spread over 3 times (3 times 3 capsules, 320 mg each) and about 8 hours apart. I also exercise — I walk or jog every day.

For me, it's a race. I've got to run long enough to get to the cure. The diet is one way to keep me running. It helps keep me focused on suppressing the disease. It's easy to become complacent since I feel fine; I can do what others do. You can't tell I have anything wrong with me.

For me, the diet is one alternative therapy, and a very important one. Diet lengthens your life. I don't expect the diet to cure me by itself. That's why I don't walk away from the medical profession or PC-SPES or alternative therapies.

My Diet Today

- My diet is basically very low fat. The only fat I use is olive oil. I shoot for a 5 to 10 percent fat diet but I know it's hard to keep that; in reality I eat more like 15 to 20 percent fat. I think 15 to 20 percent is more realistic.
- I'm not a pure vegan, but I eat very little animal fat and no dairy. I eat very little flesh. I do eat a little shrimp or calamari or occasionally a little chicken.
- I also consume about 50 to 60 grams of soy protein per day. I mix the soy isolate in a smoothie with frozen strawberries, frozen mango, frozen blueberries, and a banana. The soy protein powder is fat free.
- I eat at least 4 to 5 fruits and vegetables a day.

- I follow lots of recipes from Mike Milken's cookbooks. I use his cookbooks for two reasons: a) he tells you why you should eat certain foods; b) he makes eating interesting again. His chocolate pudding recipe is better than the real chocolate pudding.
- I take a lycopene supplement (20 mg a day) and a vitamin E supplement (800 IU) and 2 to 3 grams of vitamin C. I also take 600 mcg of selenium and a little magnesium. I take green tea capsules and I also drink green tea (a cup or two in the morning). I take saw palmetto. I look for everything that could be helpful.

I encourage men with early-stage prostate cancer to change their diet because they might be able to prevent progression of the disease without any other medical intervention. We haven't seen a cure, but we haven't had people on the diet for a long time.

There are two major points about adopting this diet: 1) In the long term it improves your quality of life. It helps suppress cancer and heart disease. 2) I think that you are able to think better when you eat these foods.

If I didn't have the disease and still adopted this diet, I would live longer and have a higher quality of life.

I think Mike Milken's efforts in prostate cancer research and his emphasis on diet have been really great. He is the leader in trying to get the world to look at the problem.

Besides following CaP CURE's nutritional recommendations, I'm a volunteer at CaP CURE. I give them one day a week for whatever they want me to do. I told them I'd even mop floors, but they haven't asked me to do that yet!

Robert Yannone

My Cancer History

I was diagnosed in 1995 and my PSA was 7.5. My Gleason score was 6. I am now 75 years old.

I decided on no treatment other than changing my diet. I've plotted my PSA every 6 months since I was diagnosed, and it has gone down.

When I was diagnosed, I visited top specialists. No one ever recommends watchful waiting. It falls in the hands of the patient to choose watchful waiting, and I chose that.

My PSA is now down to 3.9 and stabilized. Remember, I'm 75 though, so that's low; and it's still going down. I definitely think it's the diet that has lowered my PSA.

I think that diet is inseparable from the entire philosophy of health in cancer cure. I have two good chefs, my wife and daughter.

I feel good. I walk three miles every day. I may sometimes walk a little more or less.

I'm a churchgoer — I go once a week. We also have a family, and we all live together, although the house is split so that my daughter and her family can have their own space. I think it's the entire philosophy of health that counts and makes a difference.

My Diet Today

- No sugar, no salt, no caffeine. I drink decaffeinated tea and coffee.
- I avoid all hormones, including those in milk, because they could accelerate the tumor growth.
- I eat nothing that has preservatives in it.

- I eat no fat or as little fat as I can get — no red meat, a little white meat such as free-range chicken or turkey.
- I drink no liquor (one glass of wine maybe once every two weeks).
- I don't smoke cigarettes, and I avoid smoke in restaurants.
- I eat all kinds of soy products (I'll put tofu in spaghetti). I eat tofu ice cream (fat free). I eat soy yogurt. I eat tofu. I drink soymilk daily. I drink green tea.
- I eat 100 percent organic food (certified according to California law).
- I eat all types of fruits and vegetables. I eat tomatoes and tomato sauces and mushrooms — for example, shiitake and portobello. My cereals are bran cereals.
- I eat salmon once a week.
- When I eat out, I eat what I can get with an eye to what won't have preservatives.
- I take 1200 mg of vitamin C a day, 1200 mg of calcium mixed with vitamin D, vitamin E (800 IU), 200 mcg of selenium.
- Is this diet good for me? Yes, I think it is. How long will it hold? I don't know. I continue to get PSA checks and digital rectal tests. They've been fine.

Harry Pinchot

My Cancer History

I was diagnosed with metastatic disease at age 55, which ruled out a lot of options — it ruled out all local treatement, such as surgery or brachytherapy [radioactive seed implants]. It's unlikely that you can cure metastatic disease. This was in March of 1995. I was diagnosed with a Gleason score of 8 and a PSA score of 32; the PSA score was doubling every 21 to 28 days, which is very aggressive. With my oncolgist I then laid out a plan of action to be as aggressive as possible. We did simultaneous androgen deprivation therapy [hormone therapy], chemotherapy, and full pelvic radiation, which compromises your quality of life (it damages the bladder and the rectum and that changes your quality of life). We wound up with a recurrence of the disease 7 months later. We went on to androgen deprivation therapy again and added a drug which is controversial in this country, thalidomide. Thalidomide has value in certain cancers and leprosy. That started to fail me after 11 or 12 months. Then we added PC-SPES to my diet; and that worked.

We gradually increased the dose. Currently I'm on 12 PC-SPES capsules a day divided into 4 doses of 3 each, 6 hours apart (each tablet contains 320 milligrams).

My Diet Today

I changed my diet almost from the outset, in the fall of 1995. Dr. David Heber suggested a diet high in soy and with minimum fat that I've followed for 4 years now.

- My daily fat allowance is 15 grams — I usually consume slightly less than 10 percent. I don't pay attention to caloric intake; I pay attention to fat content.
- Per Dr. Heber's recommendation, which is along the same lines as Mike Milken's diet, I eat 40 grams of isolated soy protein a day. I make a shake with juice (orange juice), soy protein isolate, fruits, and anything that strikes my mood.
- I try to consume products that contain soy. We use a number of recipes out of Mike Milken's *The Taste for Living Cookbook*. You've got to love their brownies and their chocolate mousse. There's a lasagne there that's also in-

credible. There's a taco recipe that's fantastic. There isn't a single meal that doesn't have some soy in it. I try to buy all soy products fat free.

- For breakfast, I'll have cereal with fat-free soymilk or rice milk and my shake.
- For lunch, I'll eat a vegetable sandwich or a soy hamburger or a soy hot dog.
- For dinner, I'll eat whatever my wife fixes, often from Mike Milken's cookbook. She's always pushing vegetables at me.

Diet gives one a psychological sense of empowerment that you can do something that is an adjunctive therapy to the traditional medical treatment. Proactive patients survive longer than reactive patients.

The Wellness Community support groups offer yoga and tai chi as a way to help you focus your thinking. They claim benefits from meditation. There's no charge to anyone; it's all done by funding. They have several different cancer support groups. They're in most metropolitan areas: 805-379-4777.

I attended a CaP CURE conference in Tahoe. I felt very fortunate to be able to attend. I walked away with very positive feelings about both CaP CURE and Mike Milken. They're doing so many great things.

Howard Waage

My Cancer History

My first PSA test at age 46 came back at 11, but my local urologist thought it was prostatitis. He watched my PSA go up to 30. The first biopsy missed the cancer — this was at age 47. The biopsy was read improperly. I was diagnosed with prostate cancer at age 49, and my PSA was 39. It was advanced, localized prostate cancer; it had spread outside the prostate. And almost immediately after being diagnosed, I changed my diet. I got brachytherapy [radioactive seed implants] and external beam radiation therapy. I was on hormonal therapy for 6 months before the radiation and for 4 months after the radiation. My PSA is now 0.2.

My Diet Today

I am banking on my diet to keep my PSA low and to keep me healthy for a long time. Once you have eliminated the tumor burden with radiation or surgery, I think you can manage any remaining cancer with diet.

In terms of weight control and general overall health, the diet is great. It has lowered my cholesterol, my blood pressure, and my weight. And it helps keep my weight off. I feel healthier eating this way without red meat and dairy cheeses.

For men who do not have prostate cancer, diet can help prevent it. There is strong evidence showing that. It's important for someone diagnosed with prostate cancer to instruct his sons about the right way to eat, because the risk of prostate cancer doubles with prostate cancer in the family.

- I've eliminated all red meat. I eat fish. I don't eat poultry. I eat tofu products. My cereal is with soymilk. I drink lots of green tea (about 3 tea bags a day); I pour soymilk into my green tea. I don't eat any dairy. For cheese, I eat soy cheese. I eat lots of tomatoes and other vegetables and fruits and rice. I avoid fats. My only oil is olive oil.
- Supplements: I take two soy extract pills a day (megasoy extract, 135 mg per capsule). I take a selenium supplement (400 mcg a day); I take 800 IU of vitamin E a day. I take 3,000 IU of vitamin D-3 a day. I take a 1,000 mg salmon oil capsule a day. I also take a saw palmetto supplement.

- I look at labels and make sure they don't have hydrogenated oils. I stay away from safflower oil and canola oil and hydrogenated oils.
- Dr. Myers told us that dark chocolate is mainly stearic acid and that in vitro, stearic acid kills prostate cancer cells. I eat a little dark chocolate.

I eliminate as many stressors as possible from my work and my personal life. I try to redirect my focus to my family.

I do meditation — I aim for one hour a day.

It's important for men who are diagnosed to become involved in support groups. Support groups spread information.

Bill Donnelly

My Cancer History

I was diagnosed when I was 48. My father died from prostate cancer, so I was getting regular screening starting in my mid-40s. The PSA started to increase in my fourth year of testing. There was a slight increase, so I had a biopsy. The PSA at that time was 5.1, and I found that it was early cancer. My Gleason scores were 3 and 3. Two and a half years ago, in May of 1997, I had surgery. My PSA right now is 0. I had the best clinical staging and pathological scoring. Even with those good clinical conditions, 15 percent of patients relapse within 10 years. So I use diet to prevent relapse. For me, it has become a whole lifestyle change.

I'm 52 and run and snowboard and surf. I run 40 miles a week — 10 miles four times a week (but I've been running 25 years). This disease hasn't slowed me down.

I do some visualization and relaxation for 20 minutes once a day, either during lunch time or in the evening.

My Diet Today

- I have embarked on a low-fat, high-fiber diet with genistein. I keep fat content at less than 20 grams a day and fiber at 35 or more grams a day. I take 40 grams of a soy isolate powder a day. I make a shake with the powder and fruit juice and cut-up fruit.

- My diet doesn't have any red meat. I eat no fried foods and almost no dairy — no margarine, no eggs, very little oil even if it's olive oil (I might use an oil spray), and no regular salad dressing. I'll have chicken breast or some fish in a meal once a day. I eat lots of fresh vegetables and fruits and salads and grains.

- Breakfast: I'll eat a high-fiber dry cereal with a little nonfat milk.

- Lunch: I'll eat salads or a sandwich.

- I make a soy shake in the afternoon or morning, or I split the soy isolate amount in half and have 20 grams twice a day.

- Dinner: I make dinners at home — salads and steamed vegetables and some fish or chicken.

- I also take supplements of selenium (200 mcg) and vitamin E (200 IU).

- What about when I go out to eat? There are very few restaurants where you can't get what you want. I ask for grilled fish, steamed or grilled vegetables, and salad dressings on the side. We don't go to French restaurants anymore because they put a lot of cream in their food. Northern Italian food also uses a lot of cream and olive oil.

- I used to eat lots of cheese and nuts. Fried foods didn't concern me. I used to eat granola, which is high in fat. Now I don't eat any of that.

What we're talking about is a lifestyle change. For men who haven't been diagnosed and who are in their 30s and 40s, that's the time to change your diet. There is an aspect of cancer incidence that's in your control — for prostate cancer, it is strongly associated with diet and animal fat, and we know that if you change your diet and also take some supplements, you can reduce your risk. Start now to take control. People in their 30s and 40s have nothing to lose and everything to gain by pursuing this diet. They're also going to reduce their heart disease risk and cancer risk and lead a longer, healthier life with this diet.

I suggest this diet to all men, especially those who have a family history of prostate cancer and those who are African American. This diet will also be beneficial for heart disease and other cancers.

Men have to get rid of their desire for fast foods and french fries and steak and bacon and eggs — they have to turn that around. I have absolutely no desire for any of those foods.

My children (who are 16 and 13) are already learning what a good, healthy diet is. They read labels; my younger son doesn't eat red meat. They eat what I eat for dinner. They don't go to fast-food restaurants. They understand what this is about.

Appendices

Appendix One: How to Determine Your Risk of Prostate Cancer

The big three risk factors for prostate cancer are age, race, and family history. These are fixed risk factors that you cannot change. They are also the only solidly established risk factors. Once you have begun PSA testing, you will have an even better idea of what your actual risk looks like, based on your PSA test results.

Age

You may think, Hey! Of course the risk of cancer increases with age, that's true of most cancers. But what makes prostate cancer unique among cancers is that the increase in risk is exponential with age, making age the single biggest risk factor for developing the disease. The rate increases from as little as 0.3 cases per 100,000 in your thirties to well over 1,000 per 100,000 in your 60s! Look at the table on page 274 to see your risk for your age and race.

Race

Rates of prostate cancer differ sharply by race. The lowest incidence rate is recorded in Chinese living in China, followed, in ascending order, by other Asians, South Americans, southern Europeans, and northern Europeans. Men of African origin have the highest rate in the world.

Within the United States, African Americans have the highest death rate and Asians, Pacific Islanders, and American Indians the lowest. See the table on page 275.

Age-Specific Rates for Invasive
(i.e., Clinical) Prostate Cancer, by Race, 1992–1996

Rates are from SEER data. Rates are per 100,000 persons and are age-adjusted to the 1970 U.S. standard population.

Age at Diagnosis	All Races, Males	White Males	Black Males
35–39	0.4	0.3	0.3
40–44	3.8	3.3	7.9
45–49	23.0	21.0	49.1
50–54	103.0	96.6	197.6
55–59	272.7	260.8	507.6
60–64	568.2	548.9	969.8
65–69	951.1	920.9	1397.8
70–74	1255.1	1212.1	1878.6
75–79	1277.4	1211.5	1804.2
80–84	1182.4	1123.1	1551.2
85+	1079.0	1036.6	1380.1

African Heritage

In every age group, blacks have higher prostate cancer incidence rates than whites. In younger age groups, in which prevalence of prostate cancer is usually low, blacks have a much higher occurrence of the disease than whites.[1]

But what's even more alarming is that most research shows that men of African origin have more-aggressive prostate cancer. This difference may not be due to socioeconomic status or to poorer access to health care. A study conducted of men with equal-access medical care in the San Francisco Bay Area showed that blacks had poorer prostate

Incidence of Invasive
(i.e., Clinical) Prostate Cancer, by Race/Ethnicity, 1992–1996

Rates are from SEER data. Rates are per 100,000 persons and are age-adjusted to the 1970 U.S. standard population.

Race/Ethnicity	Rate 1990–1996
All races	151.9
White	147.3
White Hispanic	107.4
White non-Hispanic	150.7
Black	222.9
Asian/Pacific Islanders	81.5
American Indians	46.5
*Hispanic	102.8

*Hispanic is not mutually exclusive from whites, blacks, Asian Pacific Islanders, and American Indians.

cancer survival than whites, even with equal access to care. African-American men had a 20 to 30 percent increased death rate. These findings support other research that shows blacks having higher prostate tumor virulence.[2] Alice Whittemore, Ph.D., of Stanford University, one of the researchers on the San Francisco Bay Area study, examined whether the decreased survival could be explained by socioeconomic status. She and her colleagues linked each man's address to U.S. census data to calculate mean years of education and percentage below the poverty line. She found that while these measures had a large effect on the causes of death other than prostate cancer, they had no effect on cause of death due to prostate cancer.

Not only do blacks have higher prostate cancer mortality than whites, but data suggest there might be differences within the black race as well. A study examining the influence of place of birth on cancer mortality among black New Yorkers found that Caribbean-born men had the highest prostate carcinoma mortality rate.[3] A recent study by Dr. F. E. Glover Jr. and colleagues corroborated these findings and indicated that the highest incidence of reported prostate cancer in the world is not among African Americans but among black Jamaican men in Jamaica. And in Jamaican men, the disease was clinically more significant and lethal.[4]

The bases for these racial differences are still unknown but may be related to hormonal differences and genetic predisposition. An autopsy study of PIN lesions in blacks and whites is one of the most exciting new findings suggesting genetics might play a role.

Prostatic intraepithelial neoplasia, or PIN lesions, are premalignant lesions and are markers for the presence of cancer in the gland. The PIN lesion can be thought of as a preinvasive cancer called a cancer in situ. There are high- and low-grade PIN lesions. The higher grade shows association with prostate cancer. If a man undergoes a biopsy and is found to have a high-grade PIN in his gland, it's estimated that 40 to 50 percent of the time he will end up having a carcinoma when a follow-up biopsy is performed. Dr. Wael Sakr looked for high- and low-grade PIN lesions and examined when the lesions start and their distribution in the gland. He found more high-grade PIN among African Americans than among whites even as early as age 30.

When African Americans have high-grade PIN, they also have more-aggressive tumors. It is possible that the more prevalent high-grade PIN in African Americans could be as-

Presence of High-Grade PIN Lesions

Age	African Americans	Caucasians
30s	18%	14%
40s	31%	21%
50s	69%	38%
60s	78%	50%
70s	86%	63%

sociated with the generally more-aggressive forms of prostate cancer among African Americans. "Genetic and nutritional factors play a role," says Dr. Sakr. The deadly combination of earlier onset, increased virulence, and high death rate makes early testing critical for African American men.

Family History

A family history of prostate cancer significantly increases your risk of the disease. The most serious risk is having first-degree relatives, such as a father, brother, or son, with prostate cancer. Here's how those risks stack up. A Swedish study found that men whose fathers had prostate cancer had a 2-fold increased risk of prostate cancer. However, if men had a brother with prostate cancer, there was a 5-fold increased risk![5] If your affected relative had the disease at a young age, you're also at higher risk. First-degree relatives of early-onset prostate cancer patients had a more than 3-fold increase in the risk of developing prostate cancer before age 70 according to a Swedish study titled "The Risk of Malignant Tumors in First-Degree Relatives of Men with Early-Onset Prostate Cancer."[6]

Your risk also reportedly increases the higher the number of affected first-degree relatives you have. Alice Whittemore showed that men with a first-degree relative suffering from prostate cancer have a 2- to 2.5-fold elevated risk of developing the disease, but men who had two or more first-degree relatives with prostate cancer had a 4- to 4.5-fold increased risk if they were Asian or white and a 9-fold increased risk if they were black!

Genetics

It's not just male family members who put you at higher risk. Icelandic researchers have now found a striking relationship between BRCA2, a breast cancer gene, and prostate cancer. If you have a first-degree relative with the BRCA2 gene, you are at 4.6 times greater risk of prostate cancer.[7] Another recent study showed that in families with no history of prostate cancer, but with a family history of breast cancer, there was a modest rise in risk of fatal prostate cancer. This association was stronger for Ashkenazi Jewish men and for men under 65 with relatives diagnosed with breast cancer before age 50.[8]

The real genetic problem is for men under 55; then the genetic factors are far more prominent, contributing up to 43 percent of their risk of developing cancer.[9]

So why if you have a first-degree relative with prostate cancer are you at higher risk? Researchers are scanning the entire human genome in large, extended families to find a link between inheritance and prostate cancer. Although this research is still ongoing, three genes have already been described.

The bad news is that a family history does put you at significant risk. The good news is that only around 9 percent of total prostate cancer cases may be directly attributable to a family history of the disease, even though such a history poses a substantial risk for younger men.

Minor Risk Factors

There is some evidence that the following may be risk factors, but their importance is not as firmly established as that of age, race, and family history.

Did You Gain Substantial Weight As a Young Adult?

"Obesity and gaining weight as an adult, even as a young adult, could predict aggressiveness of the prostate tumor," says Dr. Sarah Strom, M.D., of M. D. Anderson Cancer Center. In her study, Dr. Strom examined weight gained in adulthood between the ages of 25 and 40. Men with more significant tumors also had greater weight gain, starting at age 25 and sharply increasing at age 40. Although Dr. Strom feels strongly that we can't predict individual risk based on her findings, you should carefully watch your weight for protection not only against prostate cancer, but also against several other diseases, including diabetes and heart disease.

Are You Substantially Overweight?

As of yet, there's no overwhelming evidence linking excess weight to prostate cancer risk, but in a recent study, Dr. Strom showed that a higher body mass index (the polite and scientific way of saying you're overweight!) increases risk. She compared the biomass index of men diagnosed with small prostate cancer tumors to that of men diagnosed with larger, more significant tumors. She found that men with more disease had a larger body mass index before being diagnosed with prostate cancer. The men with small volumes of tumor had a body mass index of 26 kg/m^2, whereas men with larger tumor volumes had a body mass index of 28 kg/m². The men with larger tumors had an abdominal circumference that was significantly larger, which is believed to be associated with abdominal adiposity, or body fat distribution. Men with higher tumor volumes had a higher percentage of body fat, 34 percent compared to 31 percent for men with lower-volume tumors.

If you are overweight, you'll find Part III of this book extremely helpful with its exercise, diet, and stress reduction programs.

Have You Taken Body-Building Hormones?

If you take testosterone, anabolic steroids, or other body-building hormones, you should consider at least an early baseline test for PSA. Many researchers fear that the increased hormone level puts you at risk for prostate cancer. Cells in the prostate gland are under the control of the male hormone testosterone. There's been much debate on whether men who naturally have higher levels of testosterone may also be at risk. Men who've been castrated and make very little testosterone have virtually no prostate cancer.

IGF-1

There are other hormones that you put at risk; one of the most important may be IGF-1 (insulin-like growth factor I). Since there are IGF-1 receptors on prostate cancer cells, it makes sense that IGF-1, which promotes cell growth, could attach to these receptors and make the cancer cells grow. Lab research has shown that IGF-1 strongly stimulates the growth of both normal and cancerous prostate cells. And some studies are now showing prostate cancer to be strongly associated with higher levels of the hormone IGF-1, even among men with a "normal" PSA of less than 4. Will IGF-1 become a screening test? June Chan, Sc.D., of the Harvard School of Public Health has done much of the pioneering work on IGF-1. She says, "You can measure IGF-1 in a blood sample, but we're far from a consensus about whether or not it should be used as a screening tool, like the PSA test. There is much more we need to understand about the biology of the IGF axis and prostate cancer. We also must seriously consider the consequences if we begin measuring IGF to screen for risk. What we have shown in our study is that when you compare people at the extremes of the IGF-1 distribution — in other words, the highest 25 percent versus the lowest 25 percent — then you see a 2 to 4-fold increase in risk among men with higher IGF-1 levels." (See page 320 for further information on IGF-1.)

Do You Have an Occupation That Puts You at Risk?

Studies suggest that some occupations might put you at higher risk. For example, a recent study found an unexpected significantly increased mortality from prostate cancer in men employed in the wood-cutting industry or exposed to production of those products, particularly sawdust.[10] Preliminary findings in Canada suggest that farmers and teachers may have increased risk of prostate cancer; it is not known what specific exposure may be increasing the risk, although some studies claim that the most likely explanation for the positive association between prostate cancer and farming is exposure to hormonally active agricultural chemicals.[11] It's unknown what the risk of teaching could be related to. Yet other studies show that exposure to the following substances caused a moderately strong increase in risk: cadmium, metallic dust, liquid fuel combustion products, lubricating oils and greases, and polyaromatic hydrocarbons from coal.[12] Since all of these findings are preliminary and there is no clear-cut cause and effect, consult with your doctor to see whether any new definitive findings have been made and whether your occupation might be putting you at a higher risk and warrant earlier screening.

Have You Had Bladder Cancer?

The rate of prostate cancer among men with bladder cancer is many times higher than among those without.

Have You Had a Venereal Disease?

There is a venereal disease that may increase your risk of prostate cancer. It's caused by the oncogenic human papilloma virus. You may have no symptoms, so if there's a chance you have been exposed, you may want to have your urologist investigate.

Do You Have Heart Disease?

A study from Columbia University showed that patients with coronary heart disease had double the odds of developing prostate cancer of those without. Such patients may represent a high-risk group for prostate cancer and be potential future targets for prostate cancer screening interventions.[13] The shared risk factors may be the same Western diet and weight gain associated with prostate cancer.

Are You Taller Than Six Feet Two Inches?

The ongoing U.S. Physicians Health Study, which started in 1986 in Boston, found a direct association between height and prostate cancer risk.[14] The Health Professionals Follow-up Study is a follow-up prospective study of diet and lifestyle as predictors for heart disease and cancer. Upon examining subjects in the study, Dr. Edward Giovannucci and his colleagues found that men whose adult height was six feet two inches or taller were at a 68 percent greater risk of developing advanced prostate cancer than men whose adult height was five feet eight inches or shorter.

Appendix Two: Supplementary Medical Information

Prostate cancer research is a technically advanced field, and much of the scientific writing on the subject can be pretty dense and can obscure the basic usefulness of a book like this. For those who want to know more on certain aspects of the research, I've included some supplementary information in these Appendices. The page numbers given for each entry refer to the discussion of the topic in the body of the book.

The Benefits of Lycopene (pages 101–107)

Dr. Edward Giovannucci is not alone in noting a lycopene benefit. A number of researchers have confirmed Dr. Giovannucci's findings and correlated higher lycopene serum values with decreased prostate cancer risk, and lower lycopene serum values with increased risk.[1] In their studies at M. D. Anderson, Steven Hursting, Ph.D., and his colleagues found lycopene at higher intake levels to be protective against prostate cancer risk. And Neil Fleshner, M.D., of the University of Toronto studied benign prostate tissue in patients with prostate cancer and found a decreased level of lycopene.

Second Opinion

Although an increased intake of lycopene through foods will certainly not harm you, some researchers are still not convinced that we have final proof of lycopene's benefit.

Studies by Laurence Kolonel, Ph.D., and Abraham Nomura, Ph.D., of Hawaii showed no protective benefit for lycopene in prostate cancer.

An abstract from a Finnish trial also found no relation between lycopene and prostate cancer risk.

Some experts maintain that although studies have focused on lycopene, it is perhaps other compounds in tomatoes that are linked to a decreased risk of prostate cancer. They warn that it's premature to claim that tomato lycopene is causally related to prostate cancer protection — in other words, that lycopene will actually prevent the disease. Alan Kristal, Ph.D., of the Fred Hutchinson Cancer Center in Seattle argues that it is probably antioxidation in general and not lycopene in particular that makes a difference. "Why lycopene and not vitamin C? This is the mistaken road we went down for beta carotene. Look at the literature on beta carotene and lung cancer: the evidence was much stronger than it is for lycopene and prostate cancer, and we really believed it. And then we went out and did clinical trials and found out that it's not true; not only did beta carotene not decrease cancer risk, it was shown to increase it. Beta carotene turned out to be just a marker for fruits and vegetables." The lung cancer study Dr. Kristal is referring to was a Finnish trial that showed the risk of dying of lung cancer was 4 per thousand in the placebo and about 6 per thousand a year for the group taking beta carotene — a statistically significant increase of illness with beta carotene!

Lastly, experts warn that despite Dr. Kucuk's and Dr. Wood's findings (see page 101), it's too early to claim lycopene has a therapeutic effect on an existing prostate cancer. Also, Dr. Kucuk's and Dr. Wood's study has not yet been published or undergone peer review.

The take-home message from this controversy is that you don't want to rely on lycopene supplements. You *do* want to eat tomatoes and tomato-containing foods as part of a diet rich in fruits and vegetables.

Dr. Feldman's Vitamin D Study (pages 122–123)

Here are the details of Dr. Feldman's study on vitamin D. Dr. Feldman gave 1,25-D to patients with prostate cancer. He chose patients who had had either surgery or radiation that was thought to have brought about a cure. They were not taking other drugs at the time of the study. Months or years after their treatment, their PSA began to rise. Their PSA rise was at a rate that was constant in each patient; the patient's rate of rise was linear over time — it was doubling. The goal of the study was to see if 1,25-D treatment could bend the curve of PSA rise from a steep rise to a shallow rise or even a fall. Dr. Feldman had seven patients and treated them all with calcitrol, which is 1,25-D. He varied the dose depending on the patient in order to be able to give each patient as much as he could tolerate without developing hypercalcemia (high calcium in the blood) or hypercalciuria (high calcium in the urine). Although the doses varied, Dr. Feldman says on average he could give patients 1.5 micrograms a day; he followed them over a period of 1 year and then longer. The results showed that all seven patients had a decrease in the rate of rise of PSA. The way it's described is by doubling time — in other words, how many months the PSA takes to double. In all patients the time it took to double significantly increased, from 2 months to 4, 5, or 6 months. In some cases, the PSA rose five times more slowly — for example, it went from a 4-month to a 20-month doubling time. All patients showed slowing in the rate of PSA rise. Pretty amazing, but what about side effects?

1,25-D regulates calcium absorption, and Dr. Feldman worried about causing complications such as kidney stones resulting from a rise in blood level of calcium. Sure enough, even after he adjusted the dose to avoid high calcium levels, all patients still had an increased level of calcium in the urine. Two patients developed a kidney stone. He discontinued treatment of these patients, even though the stones were small and asymptomatic. Says Dr. Feldman, "Nevertheless, we were very pleased with the results. We delayed the PSA rise for many months. Seven of 7 patients had a significant benefit; and after all, a kidney stone is not cancer." Dr. Feldman is now studying vitamin D drugs with greater potency against the cancer and reduced risk of kidney stones.

Vitamin D Analogs

Pharmaceutical companies have modified the structure of 1,25-D. These new drugs are called Vitamin-D analogs. The analogs have less tendency to raise calcium in the blood and more activity to inhibit prostate cancer cell growth. The hope is that the analog will have a wider therapeutic window. Rocaltrol, the brand name of the drug Dr. Feldman used in his study, has been on the market for several years and is used to reduce progression of osteoporosis and to treat patients with renal failure. Patients who have renal failure are treated with 1,25-D because their kidneys don't produce enough vitamin D. Rocaltrol has the potential, however, to cause hypercalcemia. Donald Trump, M.D., at the University of Pittsburgh School of Medicine is currently exploring the maximum dose for prostate cancer patients.

Genetic Risks of Developing Prostate Cancer
(pages 278–279)

William Isaacs, Ph.D., of Johns Hopkins University and Dr. Jeffrey Trent of the National Institutes of Health described two different genes that have the ability to increase the risk of developing prostate cancer. "We think that together these two genes account for from 30 to 40 percent of hereditary prostate cancer; each gene is 15 to 20 percent of risk," says Dr. Isaacs.

Most interesting was a region on the long arm of chromosome 1. Dr. Isaacs and his colleagues located a hereditary prostate cancer 1 (HPC1) locus on the long arm of chromosome 1 on position 1q24-25. Examining families with hereditary prostate cancer, Dr. Isaacs found that in the families in which men were likely to be carrying an altered HPC1 gene, the average age of prostate cancer diagnosis was lower, and the cancers were of a higher grade and at a more advanced stage of the disease.[2]

The second "increased susceptibility" region for higher risk of prostate cancer was at the 4th locus on the X chromosome: HPCX.

"At this stage we have evidence for the locations of two different genes. We have the locations but we don't know what the particular genes are for both the chromosome 1 gene and the chromosome X gene. We now need to identify the genes," says Dr. Isaacs.

Another research group, led by Dr. Elaine Ostrander in Seattle, described a third gene related to increased risk of hereditary cancer — a locus on the long arm of chromosome 1 at position 1q42-43.

What could a gene do to increase the risk? Hormones drive the growth of prostate cancer just as they do breast cancers. In fact, these two cancers are termed hormonally driven tumors. The place that hormones act to turn on a cancer are at what is called a receptor. The receptor acts like an electrical switch — it "signals" the cell to take action; for example, the receptor could tell cells to increase cell division and growth.

Of particular interest to prostate cancer researchers have been genes involved in the signaling pathway of male sex hormones, called androgens — for example, the androgen receptor gene. When Philip Kantoff, M.D., of the Dana Farber Cancer Institute in Boston and Ronald Ross, M.D., at the University of Southern California studied the androgen receptor gene, they found that when sections of the DNA code had defective "repeat sequences," the man was at a higher risk for prostate cancer. Dr. Kantoff and Dr. Ross studied repeats in two areas of the androgen receptor gene: the CAG repeat and the GGN repeat. They found that men with a family history of prostate cancer had an increased risk if they had shorter CAG repeats. And other studies have corroborated the finding that fewer CAG repeats relate to increased risk of prostate cancer. When you look at the actual DNA sequence, you'll find, as an example, the CAG genetic code in the androgen receptor is repeated between 7 and 35 times (for example, CAG CAG CAG CAG CAG CAG CAG CAG) in healthy men. When you have fewer repeats (i.e., in the lower part of this range), the risk increases compared to men in the higher part of this range. What do these repeats mean? The most interesting theory is that they change the activity level of the androgen receptor (e.g., fewer repeats would make the androgen receptor like a higher octane gasoline). They may also change the affinity of the hormone for the receptors — i.e., make it more or less sticky. You can see how these changes could either amplify or diminish the effect of androgens.

Exisulind (pages 234–235)

Researchers first gave exisulind to patients with adenomatous polyposis coli (APC). Those patients develop colon cancer early in life because they have many small polyps growing in their colon, polyps that can easily turn cancerous. After taking exisulind, the patients' number of polyps decreased — in other words, the cancer growth was slowed. From these results, researchers decided to try exisulind with other cancers, including prostate cancer.

The PC-SPES Debate (pages 235–242)

PC-SPES Ingredients

PC-SPES is made of eight different herbs — one American herb and seven Chinese herbs. Here's a brief description of each.

Saw palmetto: Saw palmetto is the American herb. Saw palmetto inhibits 5-alpha-reductase, the enzyme that is critical in converting testosterone to dihydrotestosterone (DHT).[3] European studies report beneficial effects of saw palmetto on urinary flow rates in men with benign prostatic hyperplasia (BPH). There is no proof, however, that saw palmetto has an effect on prostate cancer.

Chrysanthemum: Chinese tradition holds that chrysanthemum has detoxifying and antiviral properties.

Licorice: Licorice has some activity similar to the female hormone estrogen, as demonstrated in an estrogen-receptor-binding assay in which it competes with estradiol, the most powerful female estrogen.[4] Moreover, licorice contains saponins that in test tubes have shown antitumor activity. Licorice has anti-inflammatory and analgesic effects.

Isatis: Isatis contains the phytosterol betasitosterol, which has been shown to reduce tumor growth in animals.

Ganoderma lucidum: Ganoderma lucidum is known to have anti-inflammatory and analgesic effects. Also contains polysaccharide compounds said to inhibit cancer cells.

Panax pseudo-ginseng (from ginseng family): Researchers have speculated that this herb has estrogenic activity. Panax pseudo-ginseng is also known to have anti-inflammatory and analgesic effects.

Rabdosia rubescens: This herb is known to have anti-inflammatory and analgesic effects.

Scutellaria: Scutellaria encourages apoptosis, or cell death, so the cancer doesn't grow; also shown to have antibacterial and immune-enhancing properties.

PC-SPES Clinical Trials Results

Early-stage prostate cancer: According to Dr. Hank Portfield, the positive effect of PC-SPES on early-stage patients is independent of prior therapies.[5]

Late-stage prostate cancer (hormone-responsive): Dr. Eric Small studied 33 patients who were at late stage but were responsive to hormone therapy. He found that 100 percent of these patients showed a more than 50 percent reduction in PSA and 74 percent had a more than 50 percent decrease in tumor volume.

Progressive prostate cancer after hormone treatment (hormone-resistant): In Dr. Small's study, 37 patients had hormone-resistant prostate cancer (HRPC), meaning that hormones no longer worked. Still, even though many see PC-SPES working primarily as hormone therapy, Dr. Small also saw a drop in PSA of about 50 to 60 percent in this group. This tells us that PC-SPES has nonhormonal effects. Dr. B. L. Pfeifer reported a 70 percent reduction in PSA among his study patients, a result that is comparable to Dr. Small's finding. Both Dr. Small and Dr. Pfeifer reported that PC-SPES was well tolerated by the majority of patients. Potentially serious side effects were rare. They included allergic reactions in 4 percent of patients and blood clots that traveled elsewhere in the body in 4.3 percent of patients (thromboembolic episodes).

Second Opinions

Here is what some other researchers have to say about PC-SPES. Erik Goluboff, M.D., assistant professor of urology at Columbia University and director of urology at Columbia-Presbyterian Hospital's Allen Pavilion, says: "PC-SPES — I don't like it. It's a mixed preparation. The drug has not been tested well clinically. A few patients got heart attacks from it. The drug is not well studied."

Ralph Buttyan, Ph.D., professor at Columbia University and director of urology research says: "There is evidence, however, that this compound has an estrogenic effect which can induce heart disease in men." Despite the risk, he also says: "We've been testing it in vitro. We're finding that there's something in this drug that does kill prostate cancer cells. We don't know what exactly it is."

Patrick Walsh, M.D., professor of urology at Johns Hopkins University, says: "The effects of PC-SPES are hormonal. The major effects are hormonal and the mechanism is hormonal. The action is hormonal."

Philip Kantoff, M.D., associate professor of medicine at Harvard and director of genitourinary oncology at the Dana-

Farber Cancer Institute in Boston, says: "We don't know enough about PC-SPES to recommend it, but it has activity. PC-SPES acts more like an estrogen than a testosterone-lowering agent."

Eric Small, M.D., professor of medicine and urology at UC San Francisco, says: "PC-SPES shouldn't be accepted just because it's natural. In other words, it shouldn't be accepted on blind faith. Doctors also shouldn't just say 'PC-SPES is not going to work.' They should apply the same rigorous standard to PC-SPES as to other drugs."

IGF-1

Edward Giovannucci, M.D., June M. Chan, Sc.D., and their colleagues from Harvard and McGill Universities found that higher prediagnostic levels of the hormone IGF-1 were associated with an increased risk of prostate cancer, in an analysis of the ongoing Physicians Health Study. The association was relatively strong compared to other known prostate cancer risk factors — men with the highest IGF-1 levels were approximately four times as likely to develop cancer as men with the lowest IGF-1 levels.[6] In studies in which IGF-1 levels were measured at the time of diagnosis, it's been observed that patients with prostate cancer have significantly higher levers of IGF-1 than men without prostate cancer. In a study published by the Department of Medical Epidemiology, Karolinska Institute, Stockholm, Sweden, the authors conclude: "Elevated serum IGF-1 levels may be an important predictor of risk for prostate cancer."

Researchers are now exploring the possibility of using IGF-1 as a biomarker for subsequent prostate cancer risk, similar to how cholesterol levels are used as a warning for heart disease risk.

Finasteride and Male Sex Hormones (pages 229–233)

PSA Tracking on Finasteride

Dr. David Crawford, who studies PSA screening and is professor of urology and radiation oncology at the University of Colorado Health Sciences Center, says that PSA will read 50 percent lower in men taking finasteride. So if you're taking finasteride (sold under the trademark Proscar) to treat BPH, when you're tracking your PSA, double whatever number you are getting with finasteride. That way finasteride will not confuse the value of PSA as an early warning. The manufacturer also counters that finasteride won't interfere with a PSA tracking program. If you are taking finasteride for BPH, there may be an added benefit in terms of decreasing your risk of heart disease. That research is in its earliest stages.

Supplements That May Decrease the Sex-Hormone Levels in the Prostate

Saw palmetto: Saw palmetto is a highly popular supplement sold in health food stores and promoted for prostate health. Intriguingly, like finasteride, it is a 5-alpha-reductase enzyme inhibitor and is used by some men for BPH. However, its 5-alpha-reductase activity is considered weak and it has not been proved to be effective in the treatment of prostate cancer.

Drugs That May Increase the Sex-Hormone Levels in the Prostate

These drugs may have the opposite effect of finasteride, that is, they may further *increase* the male hormone effect on the prostate. It's not known if that increases the risk of cancer, but some urologists warn their high-risk patients against them.

DHEA: DHEA is a highly popular supplement found in health food stores. It's a male sex hormone made in the adrenal glands and has recently gained even greater popularity as a supplement for men for increasing muscle mass and energy levels and countering the effects of aging. If you have a family history of prostate cancer or are at high risk, you'll want to be extremely careful about taking DHEA, since you are adding another male hormone to your body. While we don't yet have data showing that these supplements are increasing risk, you should talk to your physician before taking such supplements. If you do take DHEA, be sure you're stepping up your PSA-tracking program.

Testosterone: The ultimate male sex hormone is available in patch or injectable form. Many men take this to increase libido and muscle mass as well as to improve youthfulness. The same warning applies here as it does to DHEA. If you want to take this drug, check with your doctor first and be sure to increase your vigilance by stepping up your PSA-tracking program.

Anabolic steroids: Body builders have been taking these for decades. As with testosterone or DHEA, you should be wary of anabolic steroids, especially if you have a family history of prostate cancer.

Male Sex Hormones and Prostate Cancer

From first principles, it would seem that male sex hormones might have a role in prostate cancer. Sex hormones may affect the progression from latent to clinical prostate cancer. Many early-stage clinical cancers appear to be dependent on male sex hormones for their growth. To test this idea, in an American and a Japanese study researchers injected androgens into rats and dogs and found that the androgen injections caused prostate cancer.

To see if this held true in humans, researchers first looked at testosterone to see if high levels were related to a risk of cancer. Ronald Ross, M.D., of the University of Southern California compared young, healthy African American men to young, healthy white men in Los Angeles. He knew there were normal daily variations in testosterone and that certain lifestyle factors affect testosterone, so these needed to be accounted for — for example, cigarette smoking increases testosterone levels, whereas alcohol can damage liver cells and lower testosterone. After taking into account these variations and subtle differences, he and his colleagues still found testosterone levels in African Americans to be about 15 percent higher than in their white counterparts; this suggested he was working in the right direction and that the assumption that African Americans, who are at a higher risk, have higher testosterone levels and Asians in Asia, who have lower risk, have lower testosterone levels might be correct. However, when Dr. Ross extended this study to examine Japanese men living in rural Japan, he was surprised to find the results did not confirm his hypothesis; in fact, the Japanese men's testosterone levels were comparable to those of whites.

Since, as we've learned, DHT is the most powerful androgen, Dr. Ross turned his attention to the risk that DHT might pose. Since he couldn't measure DHT directly in the prostate, he looked for another way. This led him to a surrogate called androstanediol glucuronide, which could be measured with a simple blood test and would indicate how much DHT was being produced. Dr. Ross found that the Japanese had low levels of androstanediol glucuronide, which meant they were not making as much DHT as white or black men. Dr. Ross's findings have been reproducible in other studies of Japanese and Chinese men in Asia. Dr. Anna Wu, Dr. Alice Whittemore, and Dr. Laurence Kolonel measured serum androgens in older men of different races and found that the amount of DHT relative to the amount of testosterone was highest in African Americans, intermediate in whites, and lowest in Asians. This provides more evidence that different races might have different 5-alpha-reductase activity, with African Americans having the highest amount of activity converting testosterone to the potent DHT.[7] This could also explain, in part, the racial differences in rates of prostate cancer. Simply put, the strongest evidence relating prostate cancer to androgens involves the hormone DHT.

Does Finasteride Work?

There are no final results to date. Here's what we know so far, what goes for and against the theory that finasteride is effective in preventing prostate cancer.

For: In the test tube the growth rate of prostate cancer cells was inhibited by finasteride. In fact, the higher the dose, the greater the inhibition.

For: Merck Research Laboratories report that following radical prostatectomy for prostate cancer, fewer recurrences were observed in the finasteride group, but these differences were not statistically significant. These data require confirmation by studies that are longer and larger.

Against: The Strang Cancer Prevention Center found that men with a PSA above 10 were not protected by finasteride — 30 percent got prostate cancer while on the drug.

Against: A short-term study from the University of Southern California's Norris Comprehensive Cancer Center, Los Angeles, concluded that there is "little evidence that finasteride is an effective chemopreventive agent for prostate cancer in men with elevated PSA."

And here are the experts' point/counterpoint arguments:

Point: Some studies have shown that the cancerous prostate contains less 5-alpha-reductase, which might mean that DHT is not so important in prostate cancer as it is in BPH.

Counterpoint: Otis Brawly, M.D., one of the investigators in the finasteride trial at the National Cancer Institute, says that DHT can be important for prostate cancer even if 5-alpha-reductase doesn't occur in prostate cancer cells. Here's why. "Five-alpha-reductase is found more in structural cells in the prostate. These structural cells are found throughout the prostate. Once 5-alpha-reductase converts testosterone into DHT, DHT can enter the bloodstream and travel from structural cells to other cells in the prostate. And DHT can travel to prostate cancer cells or to normal prostate cells, where it can promote cell growth and increase the chances of cancer."

Point: If it is testosterone and not DHT which is important in prostate cancer growth, then finasteride alone will not help and might actually hurt. How? By blocking DHT production, there may be a compensatory increase in the amount of testosterone in the prostate. This rebound could increase the risk.

Counterpoint: Says Dr. Brawley, "If we accept that there's only one androgen receptor in the prostate, DHT is ten times more potent in stimulating that receptor than testosterone. Some cancers mutate the receptor such that it becomes more responsive to testosterone than to DHT — those are more testosterone-driven cancers. So if that's true, higher levels of testosterone would drive the cancers." But, Dr. Brawley continues: "We don't buy the theory that prostate cancer is more testosterone driven than DHT driven. We have never found a prostate cancer that is clearly more testosterone driven than DHT driven. We have only found tumors in which DHT is more of an accelerator of prostate cancer growth than testosterone."

Point: Some researchers fear that because finasteride suppresses PSA readings, it might make cancer diagnosis more difficult. Finasteride *does* in fact lower PSA readings.

Counterpoint: Dr. Brawley says that the Prostate Cancer Prevention Trial is also testing whether finasteride can improve the sensitivity and specificity of the PSA test. A study by Dr. Mike Lieber at the Mayo Clinic in Rochester, Minnesota, found that finasteride decreases PSA secretion from BPH and from normal prostate tissue much more than it does for prostate cancer. Your PSA might be 4 without finasteride and 2 with it. Since 4 is the cutoff for normal, you'd miss that warning sign if you were on the drug and unaware of this phenomenon. "If we have a new cutoff with finasteride, we can improve the sensitivity and specificity of PSA," says Dr. Brawley. Giving the PSA test without finasteride, then giving a man finasteride for two weeks, and then repeating the PSA test may have diagnostic value (i.e., you can tell that if the level doesn't decrease, then it's more likely that the man has cancer). The trial is addressing the question of what are the best PSA levels or cutoffs for biospy for people on versus off finasteride?

Point: Some scientists think that some prostate cancers are androgen insensitive; and if that's true, then finasteride won't help prevent the disease at all.

Counterpoint: Hormones are actually used to treat prostate cancer. Only at a very late stage does prostate cancer become hormone insensitive.

Appendix Three:
The PSA Test Debate

How Good Is PSA As a Test?

The good news is that 70 to 80 percent of cancers are found by the test. Early clinically significant prostate cancer that is confined to the prostate gland can be detected sooner than with the old standard, the digital rectal examination. So where's the problem? In the remaining 20 to 30 percent of cases, the test comes back negative, suggesting that you don't have a tumor when you do. Another headache is the number of falsely positive tests. In as many as 70 percent of positive results, the test says you have cancer but you don't. That could lead to more tests, unnecessary biopsies, and a great deal of anxiety. Once you have a positive result, your doctor will have to use a variety of tests to determine if you have cancer or if it's just a false alarm. These begin with tests that are refinements of the PSA test (which are listed below), followed by an ultrasound examination and even a needle biopsy of the prostate.

Since there is not yet conclusive proof that early diagnosis is actually *saving* and *extending* men's lives, and since the PSA test can introduce a slew of expensive tests and surgery, all of which dramatically raise health care costs, several organizations are reluctant to recommend mass screening for prostate cancer.

Organizations that do not advocate routine or mass screening for prostate cancer include the National Cancer Institute, the American College of Physicians, the Centers for

Disease Control and Prevention, the American Society of Internal Medicine, the U.S. Preventive Services Task Force, the American College of Preventive Medicine, and the American Association of Family Practitioners. Organizations such as the American Cancer Society, the National Comprehensive Cancer Network, and the American Urological Association think that although the evidence is still inconclusive, there is enough to recommend that health care providers at least offer the PSA test to all men over age 50. This book doesn't take side in this debate but argues that knowing your PSA allows you to take protective measures and therefore is worth knowing. Let's take a closer look at why PSA screening is still hotly controversial.

Mortality Rates

The conventional wisdom is, Gee, if a screening test uncovers a cancer, then it must be a pretty good test. But for a screening test to be truly effective, it can't just find the disease — there must be some benefit to the patient, and the benefits must outweigh the harm. In the case of cancer, researchers have to demonstrate that a test reduces death and suffering. Studies have shown that mammograms will lower the death rate for women with early-stage breast cancer. However, there is no such definite proof yet for PSA testing. Sure, with PSA testing, cancers are taken out earlier, and less and less late-stage, lethal disease is seen. But talk to public-health specialists and they'll tell you that when you look at the big picture, there is no convincing proof that PSA saves lives — in other words, that it permits men to live longer than they would have had they just been diagnosed later. This isn't unusual in medicine. Cholesterol levels were lowered to reduce the risk of heart disease years before there was proof that lower cholesterol actually did reduce disease rates. Absolute proof of the effectiveness of PSA screening could take a long time if men in their fifties and sixties are having surgery for something that might not have killed them for another 10 to 20 years. Dr. Christopher Logothetis says: "Data support the idea that we haven't impacted the survival rates of the disease. That's true; however, the survival rates take 15 to 20 years to show. Prostate cancer takes 10 to 15 years to kill you."

The outcome of an illness is often dominated by the natural history of the disease; and with prostate cancer it's no different. There's a body of evidence suggesting that the natural history of prostate cancer rather than the treatment you receive is a dominant factor in the outcome — this means that even if you're treated early, you might still die at the same time you would have died had you been diagnosed later, in which case all that early diagnosis does is prolong the period during which you're called "sick." Barnett Kramer, M.D., M.P.H., of the National Cancer Institute says there are three categories of people with prostate cancer:

First, "those with fast-growing, aggressive tumors. For them, the best screening test just isn't good enough at catching the cancer before it has spread." Paradoxically, as we've seen, some of these men have low PSA levels, so PSA screening wouldn't help them. Some very aggressive prostate cancers might not reveal themselves with an increase in PSA. Why? The cancerous tissue is so abnormal that it doesn't produce much PSA. You could have a PSA of 1.5 and still have a cancer growing. In fact, Carl Olsson, M.D., chairman of urology at Columbia-Presbyterian Medical Center, warns that the most aggressive tumors have a lesser ability to produce PSA: "The Gleason score is a measure of the aggressiveness of the tumor; and high Gleason cancers generally have relatively lower PSAs." The tumor might also be made from a different kind of tissue, called neuroendocrine tissue, that doesn't make much PSA. That does beg the question: what if I started testing much, much earlier, before the cancer became so aggressive and the tissue was still normal? Researchers are looking at that question using stored blood samples. They do find that when there's a cancer, they can see an ominous fast rise, even from extremely low PSA levels, even below 1.0.

Second, "those in whom you could delay diagnosis because they have an indolent cancer that may never do any harm." Critics claim that PSA is picking up many of these latent cancers and that diagnosis introduces a cascade of negative events, causes huge negative psychological effects, and turns a "healthy" man into an anxious, "sick" one. Critics point out that the aggressive treatment of early cancers with radiation or radical prostatectomy can result in major complications, including urinary incontinence and impotence, without a proven decrease in mortality.[1] Depending on the age of the man, 50 to 100 percent of men who undergo treatment for prostate cancer will become impotent or have erectile dysfunction for at least some time after the operation; in some series of patients, 5 to 25 percent of men who undergo treatment will become incontinent and will actually wear diapers, at least temporarily. And men undergoing radiation may suffer from bowel or bladder irritability for a lifetime. Corroborative tests can help assess whether the tumor is latent or clinical. However, experts can't tell which occult tumors will progress into clinical cancers and which won't. The group of men with occult tumors poses the biggest single problem area. Although at the time of diagnosis these are "nonsignificant tumors" in view of overall longevity, who knows which of them will progress, and given the considerable aging of the American male, the years of danger are increasing by leaps and bounds. Are you being saved at age 50 from a tumor that would have killed you at age 85? The great hope is that protective measures may be proven that could keep these latent tumors quiescent for years. Generally, the indolent cancers are very low grade. The table below will give you an idea of how likely it is that your cancer could progress.

Third, "those who do benefit from earlier diagnosis and treatment." These men's tumors could grow to kill them, but when removed in time, their lives can be saved. While that would appear to be the strongest argument for PSA testing,

The Gleason Scoring System

Gleason Grade	Pathologist Reading: Kind of Prostate Cancer	Microscopic Picture: What Cancer Cells Look Like	Chance of Spreading within 10 Years
2–4	Well differentiated	Uniform shape, tightly packed	25%
5–7	Moderately differentiated	Irregular shapes and sizes	50%
8–10	Poorly differentiated	Lumped together in bigger groups. Invading connective tissue	75%

Table adapted from *The ABCs of Cancer,* by Joseph E. Oesterling, M.D., and Mark A Moyad, M.P.H.

there's much to suggest that this third category represents a minority of men who undergo testing, says Dr. Kramer. If this is the case, the PSA screening tests would indeed be ineffective in the majority of men. One study, by Dr. Thomas Stamey at Stanford University and researchers at the Mayo Clinic, indicated that of all men who have prostate cancer only 8 percent will ever feel any effects of the disease and that 92 percent of men with prostate cancer will live out their lives normally and die of other causes. According to Dr. Stamey, of the men with prostate cancer, only 3 percent or less will ultimately die of the disease.

Is There Any Evidence That PSA Testing Saves Lives?

In 1997, 41,000 men died of prostate cancer. The prediction for 1999 was that 35,000 to 38,000 men would die of prostate cancer. This could be just a fluctuation in the data or it could be early proof that PSA testing is working. A study from Olmsted County, Minnesota, does show a decrease in death rate after the introduction of the PSA test, though many experts say it's too early to conclude that testing is lowering the death rate. For instance, the Fred Hutchinson Cancer Research Center and the National Cancer Institute report: "The PSA cancer-screening test alone probably cannot explain the recent decline in deaths from prostate cancer."[2] What else could account for the decrease? Dr. Ruth Etzioni, a biostatistician at the Hutchinson Center, says, "The average man on the street should not read too much into the declining mortality numbers. What we're seeing is probably not all due to PSA testing. There are, most likely, other things going on. Other factors that may contribute to the drop include changing patterns of treatment and treatment-related deaths, or misclassification of cause of death." Still, Dr. Etzioni remains optimistic that testing will be shown to be effective. "Since we assume that PSA testing works for the individual in a clinically meaningful way, we do not address whether PSA testing is efficacious. Rather, we assume optimistically that it is, and ask instead how long it would take for this to impact the overall death rate from prostate cancer. We look forward to the results from clinical trials for more definitive answers about the efficacy of PSA testing."

The National Cancer Institute is conducting a randomized screening trial called the PLCO (prostate, lung, colon, ovary) trial to determine whether the PSA test in fact does lower mortality rates. Dr. Fritz Schroeder in Rotterdam, Holland, is also running a randomized screening trial. It will be years before the final results from these trials are in. What's the alternative? What if no screening were done at all? Sweden, where little PSA screening is done, has one of the highest mortality rates from prostate cancers in the world. If a man is diagnosed with prostate cancer in Sweden, he has a 50 percent chance of dying of it!

How Good Is PSA As a Cancer Marker?

Most experts agree that PSA is the most powerful tumor marker available in oncology today. Says Dr. E. David Crawford, "If you look at mammography, if a woman has an abnormal mammogram, she has a 20 percent chance of having cancer. If a man has an abnormal PSA and an abnormal rectal exam, he has a 50 percent chance of prostate cancer. The PSA test together with a digital rectal exam is as good as if not better than mammograms. PSA is the best, most important tumor marker available in 1999. It's good for detecting and following prostate cancer. Plus it's getting better all the time." And Dr. William Catalona adds: "Before PSA testing,

70 to 80 percent of men had incurable cancer. Now with PSA testing, 70 percent of men with a threshold of 4.0 have curable cancer; 80 percent of men with a 2.5 threshold can be cured."

The evidence seems pretty convincing, but it is still not proof positive. Researchers like to remind us early and often that PSA is still a marker and not a true endpoint. The choice is up to you. Screening alone may not be a strong enough argument, but combine PSA testing with a program of protection and keeping a report card on your progress. I would argue that if you are going to undertake a prostate cancer protection program, PSA is a great way to monitor your progress.

Backup Testing

Just having an elevated PSA doesn't mean you have prostate cancer. There are other explanations, such as age, benign prostatic hypertrophy (BPH), or even infection. While a digital rectal exam done at the time PSA is measured will help clarify the meaning of your PSA score, a number of corroborative tests have been developed to improve the diagnostic accuracy of the PSA test, lower your anxiety, and reduce the expense of unnecessary biopsies. The purpose of these tests is to clarify for men in that gray zone of PSA range from 4 to 10 who really is at a higher risk for cancer and who isn't. These tests could save you from having a biopsy.

PSA density: The PSA density measure corrects for the size of the prostate. A large prostate could account for PSA elevation. For instance, benign prostatic hypertrophy (BPH) leads to an increased prostate size and a higher PSA. PSA density is calculated by comparing your PSA level to the size of your prostate gland, as determined by an ultrasound test. So if you have a bigger prostate gland, you're allowed a higher PSA level before your PSA is considered abnormal. The overall risk of prostate cancer is higher with a PSA density above 0.15. If your PSA density is below 0.15 or remains so, follow-up biopsies are not indicated.

Age-adjusted PSA: The prostate gland grows with age, and a larger prostate means more PSA; so acceptable levels of PSA have been developed for each age range. The table below shows the generally accepted upper limits of normal values for age. Dr. Joseph E. Oesterling of the University of Michigan has determined these acceptable PSA levels for each age range. If you're in this range, he would not recommend a biopsy.

Upper Limits of PSA Values by Age and Race

Age	Whites	Blacks	Asians
40–49	2.5 ng/ml	2 ng/ml	2 ng/ml
50–59	3.5 ng/ml	4 ng/ml	3 ng/ml
60–69	4.5 ng/ml	4.5 ng/ml	4 ng/ml
70–79	6.5 ng/ml	5.5 ng/ml	5 ng/ml

Free PSA: Dr. William Catalona, who helped develop the free PSA test, says it's analogous to the cholesterol tests that help distinguish "good" and "bad" cholesterol in order to give physicians a more accurate means of studying the risk of heart disease. Dr. Catalona emphasizes that the free PSA test is helpful only for men within the PSA range of 2.5 to 10. He says: "If a man has a PSA of less than 2.5, then the risk of cancer is very low and it's hard to measure free PSA; if a man has a PSA greater than 10, then he should be biopsied regardless." The free PSA test is now FDA approved.

Here's what free PSA means: PSA exists in two forms in the blood — one form is free-floating and the other is bound to a carrier and is termed a "conjugated" form. The standard PSA test does not distinguish between the two. However, high amounts of the conjugated form are associated with prostate cancer. The free PSA test helps to distinguish between the two. Should you have a slightly elevated PSA, then doing an additional analysis to look at free PSA could help you avoid a biopsy. For example, if two men have an elevated PSA value of 6, in the patient whose PSA elevation is due to cancer, very little of that PSA is in the free form; in the patient whose PSA elevation is due to benign enlargement, more of PSA is in the free form. Says Dr. Catalona: "If the free PSA test shows more than 25 percent of free PSA, then we know we have an 8 percent chance of finding cancer in the biopsy. If the test shows less than 10 percent of free PSA, then we know we have a 60 percent chance of finding cancer in the biopsy."

PSA velocity: PSA velocity is the rate of change of PSA over time. The Baltimore Longitudinal Aging study found that in men who had a PSA that rose more than 0.75 per year, the increase was more likely due to cancer rather than benign prostatic hypertrophy. If you follow your PSA closely over time, it can be the best indication that you are heading into trouble.

Still, you'll need an expert to help you, because following this trend at very low PSA levels can be tricky. Dr. Peter Carroll of UCSF looks for a change of 0.4 or more per year.

MRI spectroscopy: MRI spectroscopy is now being used to follow patients who have prostate cancer. It differs from a standard MRI in that it looks at tumor activity. Proponents of the test say that the MRI improved considerably in those undergoing nutritional therapy and not in those in the control group. Critics say the MRI is notoriously unreliable. Dr. Walsh showed me the results of two scans of men thought to have large amounts of tumor that had spread outside the prostate. In both cases, on operation, there was very little tumor. In other words, the scan grossly overexaggerated the amount of tumor.

Ultrasound: Color ultrasound can also help doctors to decide if it's likely you have cancer. Ultrasound has made progress in leaps and bounds since the 1980s, say proponents of the technique. "Color Doppler ultrasounds have tremendous sensitivity," says Dr. Fred Lee of the Crittenton Hospital in Rochester, Michigan. They produce beautiful pictures to show the architecture of the prostate. Little cancer cells will "twinkle with color" on ultrasounds. Nearly 100 percent of ultrasounds today have color Doppler capability that will detect the new blood supply of the cancer. Little cancers disrupt normal architecture of the prostate. "We're right 50 percent of the time. If there are new blood vessels and the architecture of the gland has changed, then the positive predictive value jumps to 75 percent. Thirty-eight percent of biopsies might be avoided by proper deployment and use of these amazing new ultrasound devices. When you use a PSA of 2.5 or 3 as a cutoff, you diagnose more occult tumors, and that means more patients may go under the knife who have occult cancers. Dr. Crawford says these ultrasounds are overrated, so be sure to check with your urologist on the best follow-up course for yourself.

Any Downside to Monitoring a Prostate Cancer with PSA Tracking?

PSA tracking—great idea, you may say, but what's the downside? There is a theoretical downside for men who already have prostate cancer and are using diet, lifestyle, supplements, or drugs as a way of holding back their cancers. Let's look at the worst-case scenario. There is a concern for those who already have prostate cancer and are using nutrition as a means of treating it. The concern is that as the cancer grows and becomes more "refractory," it is harder to treat and could become more aggressive. That's an important point. Critics also worry that, used *before* surgery, a declining PSA could "mask" tumor growth, giving you a false sense of security. The biggest worry about lowering a PSA with foods or protective drugs is that PSA might *not* be a true marker for the effectiveness of prevention. In essence, the question is, could any treatment *selectively* encourage the worst cells to grow, keeping the milder cells in check, making the tumor harder to treat?

Watchful Waiting: Could a Cancer Grow without Being Reflected by an Increased PSA?

There is good preliminary evidence that a decline in PSA does mean that you have less cancer, but that is not an opinion shared by all. Dr. Patrick Walsh argues that the decline in PSA seen with any nutritional or drug therapy may simply be a decrease in the amount of PSA that the normal prostate tissue produces and does not signify any slowing in the growth of the cancer. He further argues that in the Baltimore Longitudinal Aging Study, 25 percent of men had cancers that continued to grow even though their PSAs remained level. He feels that men might be trapped by watchful waiting even if they were on a strict diet.

What you want to avoid at all costs is allowing a curable tumor to become an incurable one. You may say, "Hey, Doctor Bob, you're speaking out of both sides of your mouth! You just said PSA tracking was terrific, now you're saying it might not work so well." Well, here's the key point. You don't put yourself in a situation where your cancer does continue to grow to the point that it can no longer be cured. Even the biggest proponents of PSA tracking say that right now it is still just a theory and needs to be rigorously proved. There *is* the possibility that a more-aggressive tumor could continue to grow without showing up as a change in PSA.

PSA As a Cancer Fighter

Last, researchers at the biotechnology company EntreMed published in *The Journal of the National Cancer Institute* a paper suggesting that the body uses PSA to fight cancer by inhibiting angiogenesis, which is the blood supply that allows tumors to grow. This paper raised questions as to whether, if PSA is actually fighting cancer, the current screening method or treatment attempts that focus on lowering PSA would still be valid.

Does This Affect PSA's Usefulness As a Screening Tool?

Experts warn that the study's findings are still preliminary and that, even so, the results do not affect screening or attempts to lower PSA. William Catalona, M.D., of the Washington University School of Medicine in St. Louis, says: "This study is not going to affect PSA screening, because the issue isn't really relevant to screening. Screening looks at the relationship between high PSA and the risk of prostate cancer, and all of that research is still valid. As for the antitumor-fighting activity that they noticed, it's not really relevant because it was with astronomical PSA doses, 10,000 to 15,000 higher than you'd normally find in humans." And Dr. Crawford says, "This study does not refute PSA screening. We know that the higher the PSA, the more likely you are to have cancer. Our studies of men with advanced prostate cancer show that the higher the PSA, the less time the man lives. In one of our studies, we looked at the initial PSA scores of men diagnosed with advanced metastatic prostate cancer, and found that, on average, a man diagnosed with a PSA of less than 50 had a 4-year survival rate, for a PSA of 50 to 100 a 2.6-year survival rate, and for a PSA greater than 100 a 2.3-year survival rate." "It's a misconception to think that letting PSA rise will be beneficial, because PSA is a measure of unsuccessful control of the cancer," says Christopher Logothetis, M.D., of M. D. Anderson Cancer Center in Houston, Texas. Says Neil Fleshner, M.D., of the University of Toronto, "We know, for example, that hormone therapy knocks down PSA and extends survival. So, yes, the attempt to lower PSA is still a valid attempt."

PSA Tracking: Practical Measures

How Do I Find a Good Lab?

PSA values can vary enough to give you a pretty good scare. There is enough test-to-test variability to cause the occasional spike or dip in your PSA level. Values can vary from 15 to 20 percent, not much different from variations seen in the early days of cholesterol testing. That's because there is a substantial assay and biological variability in PSA testing. You can cut this variation down to make the test much more useful. By using a top lab at a major academic cancer center, Dr. Dean Ornish has been able to cut the variation in his tests down to just 5 percent for his current clinical trials. Most major cancer institutes are going to have very accurate labs if they are involved in prostate cancer research. You could request that your doctor send your PSA to such a lab or a lab that he or she has had solid, reliable results from. You'll want to be sure to use the same manufacturer and lab each time and that you take the proper precautions your doctor recommends before each test to prevent a spurious reading.

Since, for the purposes of this book, you want to track your PSA over time, accurate, consistent results are critical. Dr. Peter Carroll confirms that tracking PSA can be difficult to use as it requires information from several PSAs over many months to be reliable. However, followed over time, with many "points to plot," you can make this a highly useful test. If you ever charted stocks, you know that a few weeks' worth of data doesn't tell you much. You need to plot many points of data over time to see real trends. That's true of PSA as well.

One last piece of advice. In a protective program, you will probably see a drop in PSA in the first weeks with a change in food, lifestyle, medications, or supplements. That drop in PSA is probably not a decrease in tumor activity, but just a decrease in the production of PSA from normal tissue. Consider your new lower level a baseline, and watch for changes in PSA velocity. If your PSA is rising quickly within the normal range or is above 2, you may want to consider the measures in this book in combination with a more frequent tracking program. You'll want to discuss this with your urologist.

Will PSA Respond Favorably to Diet, Lifestyle, or Drug Therapy?

Yes! As you'll see, some studies have shown actual measurable declines in PSA in response to the following:

Lycopene: Lycopene decreased PSA levels by 15 percent in a group of men with prostate cancer. Those in the control group saw a 15 percent *increase* in cancer.

Fiber: In one study, fiber had the remarkable ability to actually lower PSA levels. When Neil Fleshner, M.D., assistant professor and urologic oncologist at the University of Toronto, and his associates looked at the effect of fiber intake on PSA levels, they found this direct effect: when men ate more soluble fiber, they lowered their PSA levels. Results showed that when men got soluble fiber, the PSA dropped 10 percent — a significant drop. Here are the study details:

Dr. Fleshner's was a small randomized trial with two groups and 14 men in each group. These were healthy men in their 40s and 50s — men whose PSA levels were already quite low. For four weeks, one group got 18 grams of soluble fiber and one received 53 grams of insoluble fiber; after a two-week washout, the first group got 53 grams insoluble and the second 18 grams soluble fiber. Results showed that when either group got soluble fiber, the PSA dropped 10 percent — a significant drop. Insoluble fiber had no effect on PSA. Says Dr. Fleshner: "We don't know what effect fiber would have on men with established cancers or with high PSA because we haven't studied them. This study was originally designed to look at the effect of fiber on blood lipids; but since we had the blood, we ran the PSA test — so it's a side observation. But although a side observation, it's still a real observation." The key in the study was that the fiber *had* to be a soluble fiber, which is found in oats, rice bran, certain vegetables such as Brussels sprouts and carrots, most beans, including soybeans, some fruits such as apples and oranges, and dried fruits. Soluble fiber interacts with the digestive fluids and sops up water to fill you up. Insoluble fiber — found in foods such as wheat bran, whole grains, fruits, and vegetables — accelerates the passage of food into the colon, which decreases the amount of time available to digest the food.

Genistein: Recent studies have shown that genistein (the most important component of soy) may affect PSA levels. Dr. Xiao-Ya Sun of the National Cancer Institute looked at prostate cancer cells found in lymph nodes to examine whether genistein affects the synthesis of PSA. She found that genistein inhibited the production of PSA and decreased the release of PSA.

Low-fat diet: Dr. Dan Nixon of the American Health Foundation reported to me that the right low-fat diet can actually lower PSA levels.

Drugs and supplements: In Appendix Two we look further at three drugs that can decrease PSA: finasteride, exisulind, and PC-SPES.

Stress reduction: High stress and low social support are associated with higher blood levels of prostate specific antigen, according to Dr. Arthur A. Stone and colleagues from the State University of New York at Stony Brook. Their report in the September 1999 issue of *Health Psychology* surveyed 318 men. "Men who experienced high levels of stress were more than three times as likely to have elevated PSA levels than were men who experienced low levels of stress. Similarly, low social support was nearly twice as likely to result in high PSA levels, compared to high social support."[3] Researchers are finding in preliminary clinical trials that when stress reduction is included with diet and exercise, PSA levels do drop. Without the stress reduction, there is no drop in PSA.

A Whole Lifestyle Program

Preliminary results in an ongoing lifestyle program that includes diet, exercise, and stress reduction does show a drop in PSA in men who have prostate cancer. Only those men who have at least 90 percent compliance with all three of these measures actually see a drop in their PSA. In the control group, the PSA level has continued to rise.

Ethics of Testing

Before you start PSA testing, you should consider one key ethical principle. As with all medical testing, there must be some potential beneficial result from taking a test. Quite bluntly, what do you have to gain by testing? That benefit could be psychological reassurance that you don't have cancer or it could be early curative surgery. But the test could also lead to harmful psychological turmoil based on an equivocal result or lasting negative side effects from surgery that may not have been necessary. Or, as visionaries are arguing, PSA could alert you to potential danger in time to change your diet and lifestyle and allow you to track your success.

Appendix Four: A Note for Men with Adult-Onset Diabetes

If high insulin levels are so bad for you, why don't diabetics have a high risk of prostate cancer? For those of you with diabetes, the answer is fascinating. It goes like this: While insulin resistance and its accompanying high insulin, high glucose, and high blood lipid levels might increase prostate cancer risk, once you've contracted diabetes, your risk of prostate cancer will eventually decrease. One Swedish prospective study found that prostate cancer risk increased threefold within the first year of diagnosis with diabetes, but then the risk gradually decreased over time, and 10 years after diagnosis men with diabetes had 50 percent less chance of being diagnosed with prostate cancer.[1] In another study, Edward Giovannucci, M.D., and his colleagues at Harvard examined the relationship between diabetes and prostate cancer in the Health Professionals Follow-up Study, and found that prostate cancer risk decreased in men who had been living with diabetes for over five years. The vast majority of cases that Dr. Giovannucci and his team studied were men who had adult-onset diabetes (diabetes diagnosed after age 40). Dr. Giovannucci found that prostate cancer risk increased slightly (it increased by 1.24 times) in the first five years of the diabetes diagnosis, then fell in the following five years to 0.66, and it was reduced almost by half in men who had been diagnosed with diabetes over ten years ago. You may say, Gee, how does that work? You'd expect adult-onset diabetics to have a higher risk. Well they *do*, while their insulin levels are high, but as we'll see, as the disease progresses, insulin levels fall.

Though the prediabetic state of insulin resistance produces high insulin levels, once a man becomes diabetic the pancreas can no longer produce enough insulin to keep up with the body's demand, and insulin response falls considerably. If insulin increases prostate cancer risk, then reduced insulin would mean reduced risk. Less insulin in diabetics also means less insulin-like growth factor (IGF-1), and since IGF-1 is associated with increased risk of prostate cancer, lower levels of IGF-1 would be protective.[1] Studies have shown that diabetics also have less total testosterone,[2] and since testosterone has been associated with an increased risk of prostate cancer, less testosterone could also reduce risk. Why exactly diabetes reduces testosterone is uncertain; animal studies show that diabetes is associated with fewer testicular Leydig cells (Leydig cells produce testosterone) and less testosterone secretion into the bloodstream.

Although insulin presents the most obvious explanation, scientists also hypothesize that a diabetic's change in lifestyle, for example, a change in diet, or his drug treatments might be reducing the prostate cancer risk.

Endnotes

Introduction

1. Incidence and mortality figures are from the *SEER Cancer Statistics Review, 1973–96.*

2. M. Korda, *Man to Man* (New York: Vintage Books, 1997), page 8.

3. A. I. Neugut, D. J. Rosenberg, H. Ahsan, et al., "Association Between Coronary Heart Disease and Cancers of the Breast, Prostate, and Colon," *Cancer Epidemiology, Biomarkers and Prevention* 7, no. 10 (October 1998): 869–73.

4. S. Sigurdsson, S. Thorlacius, J. Tomasson, et al., "BRCA2 Mutation in Icelandic Prostate Cancer Patients," *Journal of Molecular Medicine* 75, no. 10 (October 1997): 758–61.

5. C. Rodriguez, E. E. Calle, L. M. Tatham, et al., "Family History of Breast Cancer as a Predictor for Fatal Prostate Cancer," *Epidemiology* 9, no. 5 (September 1998): 525–9.

6. N. Walach, I. Novikov, I. Milievskaya, et al., "Cancer Among Spouses: Review of 1995 Couples," *Cancer* 82 (January 1, 1998): 180–5.

PART I: A NUTRITIONAL DISEASE

1. M. J. Hill, "Nutrition and Human Cancer," *Annals of the New York Academy of Science* 833 (December 29, 1997): 68–78.

2. *Nutrition and Prostate Cancer: A Monograph from the CaP CURE Nutrition Project,* third edition, January 1999, page 4.

3. Ibid., page 7.

PART II

Soy

1. J. R. Herbert, T. G. Hurley, B. C. Olendzki, et al., "Nutritional and Socioeconomic Factors in Relation to Prostate Cancer

Mortality: A Cross-National Study," *Journal of the National Cancer Institute* 90, no. 21 (November 4, 1998): 1637–47.

Fats

1. R. Hayes, "Dietary Factors and Risk for Prostate Cancer Among Blacks and Whites," *Cancer Epidemiology, Biomarkers and Prevention* (January 1999).

2. E. Giovannucci, E. B. Rimm, G. A. Colditz, et al., "A Prospective Study of Dietary Fat and Risk of Prostate Cancer," *Journal of the National Cancer Institute* 85, no. 19 (October 6, 1993): 1571–9.

3. J. Ghosh, C. E. Myers, "Inhibition of Arachidonate 5-Lipoxygenase Triggers Massive Apoptosis in Human Prostate Cancer Cells," *Proceedings of the National Academy of Sciences of the U.S.A.* 95, no. 22 (October 27, 1998): 13182–7.

4. P. A. Godley, M. K. Campbell, P. Gallagher, et al., "Biomarkers of Essential Fatty Acid Consumption and Risk of Prostatic Carcinoma," *Cancer Epidemiology, Biomarkers and Prevention* 5, no. 11 (November 1996): 889–95.

5. S. Harvei, K. S. Bjerve, S. Tretli, et al., "Prediagnostic Level of Fatty Acids in Serum Phospholipids: Omega-3 and Omega-6 Fatty Acids and the Risk of Prostate Cancer," *International Journal of Cancer* 71, no. 4 (May 16, 1997): 545–51.

Antioxidants

1. In one study, androgen stimulation in prostate cancer cells increased oxidation and oxidative stress. See M. O. Ripple, W. F. Henry, R. P. Rago, et al., "Prooxidant-Antioxidant Shift Induced by Androgen Treatment of Human Prostate Carcinoma Cells," *Journal of the National Cancer Institute* 89 (1997): 40–48.

2. T. Chisaka, et al., *Chemical and Pharmaceutical Bulletin,* Tokyo, 1988.

3. C. S. Yang, Z. Y. Wang, "Tea and Cancer," *Journal of the National Cancer Institute* 38 (1993): 1049–58.

4. J. W. Fahey, Y. Zhang, P. Talalay, "Broccoli Sprouts: An Exceptionally Rich Source of Inducers of Enzymes That Protect

against Chemical Carcinogens," *Proceedings of the National Academy of Sciences of the U.S.A.* 94 (September 1997): 10367–72.

5. *Wall Street Journal,* December 10, 1999, B1, "Popping Megavitamins May Sabotage Therapy to Eradicate Cancer."

Lycopene

1. E. Giovannucci, A. Ascherio, E. B. Rimm, et al., "Intake of Carotenoids and Retinol in Relation to Risk of Prostate Cancer," *Journal of the National Cancer Institute* 87, no. 23 (December 6, 1995): 1767–76.

2. P. Di Mascio, S. Kaiser, H. Sies, "Lycopene as the Most Efficient Biological Carotenoid Singlet Oxygen Quencher," *Archives of Biochemistry and Biophysics* 274 (1989): 532–8.

Starches and Sugars

1. D. M. Peehl, T. A. Stamey, "Serum-free Growth of Adult Human Prostatic Epithelial Cells," *In Vitro Cellular and Developmental Biology* — Animal Journal 22 (1986): 82–90.

2. L. Chatenoud, A. Tavani, C. La Vecchia, et al., "Whole-Grain Food Intake and Cancer Risk," *International Journal of Cancer* 77, no. 1 (July 3, 1998): 24–8; J. R. Hebert, T. G. Hurley, B. C. Olendzki, et al., "Nutritional and Socioeconomic Factors in Relation to Prostate Cancer Mortality: a Cross-National Study," *Journal of the National Cancer Institute* 90, no. 21 (November 4, 1988): 1637–47.

3. E. A. Lew, L. Garfinkel, "Variations in Mortality by Weight among 750,000 Men and Women," *Journal of Chronic Diseases* 32 (1979): 563–76.

4. P. K. Mills, W. L. Beeson, R. L. Phillips, et al., "Cohort Study of Diet, Lifestyle, and Prostate Cancer in Adventist Men," *Cancer* 64 (1989): 598–604.

Fiber

1. L. Chatenoud, A. Tavani, C. La Vecchia, et al., "Whole Grain Food Intake and Cancer Risk," *International Journal of Cancer* 77, no. 1 (July 3, 1998): 24–8; D. R. Jacobs, Jr., L. Marquart, J. Slavin, et

al., "Whole-Grain Intake and Cancer: An Expanded Review and Meta-Analysis," *Nutrition and Cancer* 30, no. 2 (1998): 85–96.

2. L. Thompson, "Antioxidants and Hormone-Mediated Health Benefits of Whole Grains," *Critical Reviews in Food Science and Nutrition* 34, nos. 5, 6 (1994): 473–97.

PART III
Stress

1. J. K. Kiecolt-Glaser, W. Garner, C. E. Speicher, et al., "Psychosocial Modifiers of Immunocompetence in Medical Students," *Psychosomatic Medicine* 46 (1984): 7–14.

2. J. K. Kiecolt-Glaser, W. B. Malarkey, M. Chee, et al., "Negative Behavior During Marital Conflict Is Associated with Immunological Down-Regulation," *Psychosomatic Medicine* 55 (1993): 395–409.

3. J. K. Kiecolt-Glaser, R. Glaser, J. T. Cacioppo, et al., "Marital Conflict in Older Adults: Endocrinological and Immunological Correlates," *Psychosomatic Medicine* 59 (1997): 339–49.

4. J. K. Kiecolt-Glaser, J. R. Dura, C. E. Speicher, et al., "Spousal Caregivers of Dementia Victims: Longitudinal Changes in Immunity and Health," *Psychosomatic Medicine* 53 (1991): 345–62.

5. J. K. Kiecolt-Glaser, P. T. Marucha, W. B. Malarkey, et al., "Slowing of Wound Healing by Psychological Stress," *Lancet* 346 (November 4, 1995): 1194–6.

6. R. Glaser, J. K. Kiecolt-Glaser, P. T. Marucha, et al., "Stress-Related Changes in Proinflammatory Cytokine Production in Wounds," *Archives of General Psychiatry* 56 (May 1999): 450–6.

7. R. Glaser, J. K. Kiecolt-Glaser, R. H. Bonneau, et al., "Stress-Induced Modulation of the Immune Response to Recombinant Hepatitis B-Vaccine," *Psychosomatic Medicine* 54 (1992): 22–9.

8. J. K. Kiecolt-Glaser, R. Glaser, S. Gravenstein, et al., "Chronic Stress Alters the Immune Response to Influenza Virus Vaccine in Older Adults," *Proceedings of the National Academy of Sciences of the U.S.A.* 93 (April 1996): 3043–7.

9. J. K. Kiecolt-Glaser, R. Stephens, P. Lipitz, et al., "Distress and DNA Repair in Human Lymphocytes," *Journal of Behavioural*

Medicine 8 (1985): 311–20; R. Glaser, B. E. Thorn, K. L. Tarr, et al., "Effects of Stress on Methyltransferase Synthesis: An Important DNA Repair Enzyme," *Health Psychology* 4 (1985): 403–12; L. D. Tomei, J. K. Kiecolt-Glaser, S. Kennedy, R. Glaser, "Psychological Stress and Phorbol Etser Inhibition of Radiation-Induced Apoptosis in Human PBLs," *Psychiatry Research* 33 (1990): 59–71.

10. R. A. Hummer, R. G. Rogers, C. B. Nam, et al., "Religious Involvement and U.S. Adult Mortality," *Demography* 36, no. 2 (May 1999): 273–85.

11. H. G. Koenig, et al., "Does Religious Attendance Prolong Survival? A Six-Year Follow-up Study of 3,968 Older Adults," *Journal of Gerontology* 54A (July 1999): 370–7.

12. McClure and Loden, 1982.

13. H. G. Koenig, L. K. George, H. J. Cohen, et al., "The Relationship between Religious Activities and Blood Pressure in Older Adults," *International Journal of Psychiatry in Medicine* 28 (February 1998): 189–213.

14. H. G. Koenig, D. B. Larson, "Use of Hospital Services, Religious Attendance, and Religious Affiliation," *Southern Medical Journal* 91 (October 1998): 925–32.

15. B. G. Berger, D. R. Owen, "Mood Alteration with Yoga and Swimming: Aerobic Exercise May Not Be Necessary," *Perceptual and Motor Skills* 75 (1992): 1333.

Exercise

1 I. M. Lee, R. S. Paffenbarger, Jr., C. C. Hsieh, "Physical Activity and Risk of Prostatic Cancer Among College Alumni," *American Journal of Epidemiology* 135 (1992): 169–75.

2. A. C. Hackney, "The Male Reproductive System and Endurance Exercise," *Medicine and Science in Sports and Exercise* 28 (1996): 180–9.

3. T. Busso, K. Häkkinen, A. Pakarinen, et al., "Hormonal Adaptations and Modelled Responses in Elite Weightlifters during 6 Weeks of Training," *European Journal of Applied Physiology and Occupational Physiology* 64 (1992): 381–6; K. Häkkinen, A.Pakarinen, M. Alen, et al., "Relationships between Training Vol-

ume, Physical Performance Capacity, and Serum Hormone Concentrations during Prolonged Training in Elite Weight Lifters," *International Journal of Sports Medicine* 8 (1987; Suppl. 1): 61–5; G. D. Wheeler, M. Singh, W. D. Pierce, et al., "Endurance Training Decreases Serum Testosterone Levels in Men without Change in Luteinizing Hormone Pulsatile Release," *Journal of Clinical Endocrinology and Metabolism* 72 (1991): 422–5.

4. M. S. Hovenanian, C. D. Deming, "The Heterologous Growth of Cancer of the Human Prostate," *Surgery Gynecology and Obstetrics* 86 (1948): 29–35.

5. P. H. Gann, C. H. Hennekens, J. Ma, et al., "A Prospective Study of Sex Hormone Levels and Risk of Prostate Cancer," *Journal of the National Cancer Institute* 88 (1996): 1118–26.

6. P. H. Gann, M. L. Daviglus, A. R. Dyer, et al., "Heart Rate and Prostate Cancer Mortality: Results of a Prospective Analysis," *Cancer Epidemiology, Biomarkers and Prevention* 4 (1995): 611–16.

7. D. Albanes, A. Blair, P. R. Taylor, "Physical Activity and Risk of Cancer in the NHANES I Population," *American Journal of Public Health* 79 (1989): 744; R. C. Brownson, J. C. Chang, J. R. Davis, et al., "Physical Activity on the Job and Cancer in Missouri," *American Journal of Public Health* 81 (1991): 639; J. E. Vena, S. Graham, M. Zielezny, et al., "Occupational Exercise and Risk of Cancer," *American Journal of Clinical Nutrition* 45 (1987): 318.

8. R. K. Severson, A. M. Nomura, J. S. Grove, et al., "A Prospective Analysis of Physical Activity and Cancer," *American Journal of Epidemiology* 130 (1989): 522; H. Yu, R. E. Harris, E. L. Wynder, "Case-Control Study of Prostate Cancer and Socioeconomic Factors," *Prostate* 13 (1988): 317; R. S. J. Paffenbarger, R. T. Hyde, A. L. Wing, "Physical Activity and Incidence of Cancer in Diverse Populations: A Preliminary Report," *American Journal of Clinical Nutrition* 45 (Suppl.) (1987): 312; A. P. Polednak, "College Athletics, Body Size, and Cancer Mortality," *Cancer* 38 (1976): 38.

9. Jane L. Harte, Georg H. Eifert, "The Effect of Running, Environment, and Attentional Focus on Athletes' Catecholamine and Cortisol Levels and Mood," *Psychophysiology* 32 (1995): 49–54.

PART IV: PROTECTION
Early Warning: The PSA Test

1. R. A. Stephenson, J. L. Stanford, "Population-Based Prostate Cancer Trends in the United States: Patterns of Change in the Era of Prostate-Specific Antigen," *World Journal of Urology* 15, no. 6 (1997): 331–5.

APPENDIX ONE:
HOW TO DETERMINE YOUR RISK OF PROSTATE CANCER

1. R. M. Merrill, D. L. Weel, E. J. Feuer, "The Lifetime Risk of Developing Prostate Cancer in White and Black Men," *Cancer Epidemiology, Biomarkers and Prevention* 6, no. 10 (October 1997): 763–8.

2. A. S. Robbins, A. S. Whittemore, S. K. Van Den Eeden, "Race, Prostate Cancer Survival, and Membership in a Large Health Maintenance Organization," *Journal of the National Cancer Institute* 90, no. 13 (July 1, 1998): 986–90.

3. J. Fang, S. Madhavan, M. H. Alderman, "Influence of Nativity on Cancer Mortality among Black New Yorkers," *Cancer* 80, no. 1 (July 1, 1997): 129–35.

4. F. E. Glover, Jr., D. S. Coffey, L. L. Douglas, et al., "The Epidemiology of Prostate Cancer in Jamaica," *Journal of Urology* 159, no. 6 (June 1998): 1984–6.

5. S. O. Andersson, J. Baron, R. Bergstrom, et al., "Lifestyle Factors and Prostate Cancer Risk: A Case-Control Study in Sweden," *Cancer Epidemiology, Biomarkers and Prevention* 5, no. 7 (July 1996): 509–13.

6. O. Bratt, U. Kristoffersson, R. Lundgren, et al., "The Risk of Malignant Tumors in First-Degree Relatives of Men with Early Onset Prostate Cancer: A Population-Based Cohort Study," *European Journal of Cancer* 33, no. 13 (November 1997): 2237–40.

7. S. Sigurdsson, S. Thorlacius, J. Tomasson, et al., "BRCA2 Mutation in Icelandic Prostate Cancer Patients," *Journal of Molecular Medicine* 75, no. 10 (October 1997): 758–61.

8. C. Rodriguez, E. E. Calle, L. M. Tatham, et al., "Family History of Breast Cancer as a Predictor for Fatal Prostate Cancer," *Epidemiology* 9, no. 5 (September 1998): 525–9.

9. E. Giovannucci, "How Is Individual Risk for Prostate Cancer Assessed?" *Hematology and Oncology Clinics of North America* 10, no. 3 (June 1996): 537–48.

10. S. D. Stellman, P. A. Demers, D. Colin, et al., "Cancer Mortality and Wood Dust Exposure among Participants in the American Cancer Society Cancer Prevention Study-II (CPS-II)," *American Journal of Industrial Medicine* 34, no. 3 (September 1998): 229–37.

11. J. A. Buxton, R. P. Gallagher, N. D. Le, et al., "Occupational Risk Factors for Prostate Cancer Mortality in British Columbia, Canada," *American Journal of Industrial Medicine* 35, no. 1 (January 1999): 82–6; J. E. Keller-Byrne, S. A. Khuder, E. A. Schaub, "Meta-analyses of Prostate Cancer and Farming," *American Journal of Industrial Medicine* 31, no. 5 (May 1997): 580–6.

12. K. J. Aronson, J. Siemiatycki, R. Dewar, et al., "Occupational Risk Factors for Prostate Cancer: Results from a Case-Control Study in Montreal, Quebec, Canada," *American Journal of Epidemiology* 143, no. 4 (February 15, 1996): 363–73.

13. A. I. Neugut, D. J. Rosenberg, H. Ahsan, et al., "Association between Coronary Heart Disease and Cancers of the Breast, Prostate, and Colon," *Cancer Epidemiology, Biomarkers and Prevention* 7, no. 10 (October 1998): 869–73.

14. E. Giovannucci, E. B. Rimm, M. J. Stampfer, et al., "Height, Body Weight, and Risk of Prostate Cancer," *Cancer Epidemiology, Biomarkers and Prevention* 6, no. 8 (August 1997): 557–63; P. R. Hebert, U. Ajani, N. R. Cook, et al., "Adult Height and Incidence of Cancer in Male Physicians," *Cancer Causes and Control* 8, no. 4 (July 1997): 591–7.

APPENDIX TWO: SUPPLEMENTARY MEDICAL INFORMATION

1. S. K. Clinton, C. Emenhiser, S. J. Schwartz, et al., "Cis-trans Lycopene Isomers, Carotenoids, and Retinol in the Human Prostate," *Cancer Epidemiology, Biomarkers and Prevention* 5, no. 10 (October 1996): 823–33.

2. H. Gronberg, S. D. Isaacs, J. R. Smith, et al., "Characteristics of Prostate Cancer in Families Potentially Linked to the Hereditary

Prostate Cancer 1 (HPC1) Locus," *Journal of the American Medical Association* 278, (October 15, 1997): 1251–5.

3. R. S. DiPaola, et al., "Clinical and Biologic Activity of an Estrogenic Herbal Combination (PC-SPES) in Prostate Cancer," *New England Journal of Medicine* 339, no. 12 (September 17, 1998): 785–91.

4. Ibid.

5. H. Portfield, "Prostate Cancer Survivors Support Groups, Survey of Us Too Members and Other Prostate Cancer Patients to Evaluate the Efficacy of PC-SPES as Well as Toxicity and Side Effects, if Any," *Molecular Urology* 3, no. 3 (1999): 333–5.

6. J. M. Chan, M. J. Stampfer, E. Giovannucci, et al., "Plasma Insulin-like Growth Factor-I and Prostate Cancer Risk: A Prospective," *Science* 279 (January 23, 1998): 563–5.

7. A. H. Wu, A. S. Whittemore, L. N. Kolonel, et al., "Serum Androgens and Sex Hormone-Binding Globulins in Relation to Lifestyle Factors in Older African-American, White, and Asian Men in the United States and Canada," *Cancer Epidemiology, Biomarkers and Prevention* 4 (October–November 1995): 735–41.

APPENDIX THREE: THE PSA TEST DEBATE

1. M. L. Lefevre, "Prostate Cancer Screening: More Harm Than Good?" *American Family Physican* 58, no. 2 (August 1998): 432–8.

2. Press release, June 15, 1999.

APPENDIX FOUR: A SPECIAL NOTE FOR MEN WITH DIABETES

1. H. O. Adami, J. McLaughlin, A. Ekbom, et al., "Cancer Risk in Patients with Diabetes Mellitus," *Cancer Causes and Control* 2 (1991): 307–14.

2. L. A. Back, M. M. Rechler, "Insulin-like Growth Factors and Diabetes," *Diabetes Metabolism Reviews* 8 (1992): 229–57.

Index